the pilates
difference

the pilates

difference

Jennifer Dufton

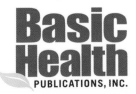

Basic Health
PUBLICATIONS, INC.

Jennifer Dufton is a fully qualified Pilates teacher and has a Pilates studio in North Norfolk. Before moving to Norfolk, she taught Pilates in some of London's most prestigious studios including the Chelsea Harbour Club, Triyoga in Primrose Hill, the Pilates Studio in Great Portland Street, and the Westminster Physiotherapy Centre. She has worked with a wide range of clients including actors, models, musicians, and members of the Royal Ballet. She is a member of The PILATESfoundation® UK, having trained with one of its co-founders, Anne-Marie Zulkahari. She also qualified with Alan Herdman Studios, and with the International Body Arts and Science Teacher Training Program under Rael Isacowitz.

First published in North America in 2004
by Basic Health Publications, Inc.
First published 2003 in Great Britain
under the title PILATES DIFFERENCE
by Hamlyn (an imprint, part of) Octopus Group Ltd.
2–4 Heron Quays, Docklands, London E14 4JP

Basic Health Publications, Inc.

8200 Boulevard East
North Bergen, NJ 07047
1-800-575-8890

ISBN: 1-59120-116-0

Printed in the United States of America

10 9 8 7 6 5 4 3 2 1

contents

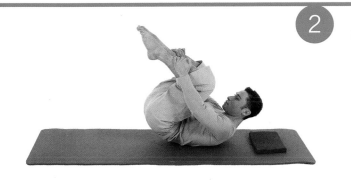
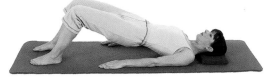
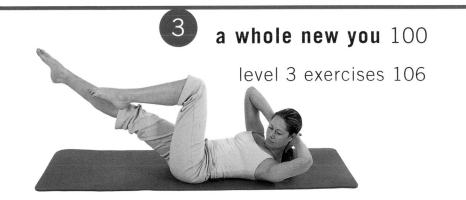

the Pilates method

Imagine you could get a great body, grow taller, improve your strength and flexibility, improve your posture, relieve aches and pains, improve your sex life, decrease stress, and boost your energy and confidence all through one kind of exercise. Better still, imagine that you actually enjoy doing it.

If your usual approach to fitness begins by looking at your body in disgust, then hurling yourself into a wild cardiovascular frenzy in order to lose the extra weight, or spending hours in the gym to tone up flabby areas, then help is at hand. Even if your chosen exercise method has the potential to work in the long term, you never find out, because you're never able to keep it up long enough. It is too exhausting and too boring. Your routine becomes yet another arduous task to be ticked off the list at the end of the day. You aren't enjoying the process so you give it up and go back to your old couch-potato ways.

The Pilates Difference is exactly what it says it is, *different*. Instead of being a mindless exercise, Pilates is one in which you have to engage your mind, which means you don't get bored. Every time you do a Pilates session, it feels fresh and new. Better still, it is extremely relaxing and you come out of the session feeling great. How many times have you walked out of the gym feeling exhausted or come in from a run and collapsed in a heap on the sofa? After a Pilates session, you don't feel wiped out. Quite the opposite. You feel rested, revitalized, years younger.

starting Pilates

This book features a program of mat-based Pilates exercises that you can use to take your first thirty Pilates lessons. It is aimed at adults of all ages, men and women, and suitable for all levels of fitness. You'll work at your own pace, tailoring exercises to suit your individual needs.

what pilates can do for you

- Give you the flexibility gained from yoga.

- Give you the muscle work of weight training without bulking up your body.

- Give you a strong, toned body, with a flatter stomach, longer, leaner muscles, and a more streamlined shape.

- Improve your posture.

- Relieve many aches and pains.

- Give you an extraordinary feeling of well-being.

- Decompress your spine so you may even regain lost height.

caution

Since you are doing the exercises at home by yourself, you need to be in good health with no injuries or medical conditions that would prevent you from undertaking the program. If you have any doubts, check with your doctor first, and also consult a qualified Pilates instructor in case any of the exercises are unsuitable for your condition.

Joseph Pilates

Joseph Pilates is the man behind the Pilates method, of which he made the following claim:

"In 10 sessions, you will feel the difference, in 20 you will see the difference, and in 30 you'll have a whole new body."

Born near Dusseldorf in Germany in 1880, Joseph Pilates was a sickly child and suffered from asthma, rickets, and rheumatic fever. However, he refused to be limited by his illnesses and, even though he was only a young boy, determined to improve his physical condition. He threw himself into a program of body conditioning and achieved such good results that by the age of 14 he was posing as a model for anatomical drawings.

He went on to become a gymnast, a boxer, and even a circus performer. He also became a devotee of yoga and martial arts. It was his continued determination to cure his own body and improve the health of those around him that led to his researching and developing an entirely new exercise regimen in the early 1900s, which he termed "Contrology." Contrology combined Eastern and Western approaches and was a program specifically designed to control the muscles by using the mind.

In 1912, Joseph Pilates moved to England where he taught self-defence to detectives at Scotland Yard, but when the First World War broke out, he was interned as a German national. He used his enforced leisure to refine his exercise method and began teaching his program of mat-based exercises to fellow internees.

During the latter part of the war, Joseph Pilates worked on the Isle of Man as an orderly in a hospital where he began working with patients who were unable to walk. He devised exercise equipment for his patients by attaching springs to hospital beds to provide resistance, and found his patients recovered more speedily than those not under his care. These spring-based pieces of equipment became the prototypes for the machines that he would later design for his equipment-based studios in New York.

After the war, Joseph Pilates returned briefly to Germany where he worked as a trainer to the Hamburg Police force. In 1926 he emigrated to the United States. On the voyage over, he met his future wife, a nurse called Clara, and by the end of the trip, they had decided to open the first official Pilates Studio in New York City. The Pilates studio was an immediate success as it became the secret of New York's finest ballet dancers and athletes.

practicing Pilates today

Since the 1920s, the popularity of Pilates has been steadily growing, and today it is a worldwide phenomenon. Popular with anyone wanting a strong and flexible body, it is also highly acclaimed by osteopaths, chiropractors, and surgeons for being safe and extremely effective. Pilates mat-classes can be found worldwide, and Pilates equipment studios are now widely available for rehabilitation work, or for those simply wanting to take this remarkable exercise method one step further.

The technique has developed somewhat over the decades, with many instructors adapting some of Joseph Pilates' original exercises according to new thinking on physical alignment and in order to modify them for all levels of fitness.

mind and body benefits

Pilates is different. So leave all your preconceptions about exercise at the door, and open your mind to a whole new way of moving.

mind–body connection

Pilates is a holistic method, drawing from both Eastern and Western philosophies. It requires you to focus your mind on individual muscles in your body so as to strengthen and lengthen them. As you move, this concentration and precision creates a mind–body connection. The additional mental focus means the muscles work to the maximum, so you get better, quicker results. Forming a mind–body connection is used to great effect in professional sport, for example, where just by shifting mental focus, a very good player can become an outstanding player. Pilates can give you that same mental breakthrough, which will then allow your body to get into the best physical shape it can possibly be.

develop a toned, lean body

✓ Saddlebag thighs slim down.

✓ Stomach becomes firmer and flatter.

✓ Waistline shrinks, the buttocks lift and tighten.

✓ Wobbly arms become firmer and leaner.

Pilates will increase your muscle strength and give you better muscle definition. Unlike many other forms of exercise, which tend to concentrate on just the superficial muscles of the body, Pilates works the deeper muscles, too, so the whole body gets a balanced workout. And unlike exercise programs that can cause the muscles to shorten and bulk up, giving you a chunky look, Pilates lengthens the muscles so that your body shape becomes more streamlined.

Pilates works to build what is known as **Functional Strength**. This means building as much strength in the body as you can, without sacrificing flexibility, and therefore good body alignment. To take it to the extremes, if you concentrate on building massive body strength without looking at the other implications, you may find you have enough strength to lift a car, but your muscle bulk means you can't bend over to touch your toes or comfortably lift your arms above your head. Pilates builds just the right amount of muscle that your body needs and that you are likely to use in everyday life. Think more of Jackie Chan's lean strength and agility than The Terminator's bulk and stiffness.

improve your flexibility

✓ Stretch out all your muscles.

✓ Lubricate your stiff joints.

✓ Allow your body to move more freely.

✓ Reduce aches and pains.

✓ Move more comfortably in daily life.

Nowadays, many of us lead fairly inactive lives spending the best part of our day sitting down, maybe slumped at a desk, or collapsed on the sofa at home. Even if you do go to the gym, do you tend to concentrate on the muscle building part of your program, and then skip the stretches afterward in your dash for the shower? Habits like these can often lead to stiffness in your body, making you more inflexible as the years pass.

Prolonged sitting in poor posture will usually cause your abdominals to weaken, the muscles in the backs of your legs to shorten, your spine to slump, and your shoulders to round forward. This can lead to lower backache, and chronic neck and shoulder pain. If you are spending long periods sitting badly, the chances are you need to improve your posture and your flexibility.

A well-moving joint is a well-lubricated joint. When your joint moves, it releases synovial fluid, which works like oil on a rusty hinge. When you do Pilates exercises in a slow, controlled manner, you increase synovial fluid production, whether it is in the spine, hips, shoulders, or elbows. This keeps your joints flexible, protects them from seizing up and decreasing your range of movement, and may help to prevent arthritis.

Pilates aims to improve what is known as **Functional Flexibility**. This means getting as flexible as you can be, without sacrificing muscle strength and therefore good alignment in the process. To perform at its best, your body needs **optimum Functional Flexibility** and **optimum Functional Strength**. No more, and no less. This is very different from many other exercise regimes and aims to keep your body perfectly balanced.

better body alignment

In addition to sitting in poor posture, are you using the same muscles over and over again? Do you always hold a telephone with the same hand or carry your shoulderbag or briefcase on the same side? Repetitive movements affect the symmetry of your body so that you become more developed on one side than the other. Your body may fall into bad patterns of behavior, which can affect your posture and muscle balance and lead to aches and pains. Pilates rebalances your muscles for better body alignment and, in doing so, improves your posture.

postural benefits

- **Weak muscles become strong.**
- **Chronically overused muscles learn to relax.**
- **Rounded shoulders begin to open and drop down.**
- **Collapsed stomach muscles lift and strengthen to support your spine.**
- **A slumped spine lengthens and straightens.**
- **A rigid spine softens and regains its natural curves.**

less stress, more vitality

If your life seems to grow ever more stressful, you need to manage stress better if it is not to control your life. With Pilates, the combination of focusing your mind, breathing well, and relaxing and moving your body greatly reduces the effects of stress. Many people also find their blood pressure lowers through regular Pilates practice.

View your Pilates practice as a safe haven. Use your sessions to grab some time for yourself, to unwind, de-stress, and revive. When you finish, you'll feel relaxed, reinvigorated, more grounded, and ready to face new challenges.

healing with pilates

Your body stores all your emotions, whether good or bad, and this affects your posture. You hold your body differently when you are happy from when you are sad or angry and if you sustain a particular emotion for a long time, your body may retain that posture. For example, if someone feels a need to be protected, they may frequently round their shoulders forward to protect their center. Over time, their pectoral muscles become short and tight, resulting in a permanently round-shouldered posture. Learning to be aware of your body doesn't just mean learning how it moves, but also how it feels.

Through trauma, apathy, or neglect, your muscles can lose their strength, ligaments lose their elasticity, and connective tissue hardens. Since Pilates calls upon the mind to move muscles with precision, it can help you to become more aware of the subtle connection between body and mind. By releasing our bodies through exercise, perhaps we can also heal our minds.

increase mental alertness

Breathing well improves the quality of your blood supply and therefore your level of alertness. By breathing well in Pilates, you will clear your mind and leave it more able to take in and process new information. In Pilates exercises you are often coordinating complex movement. This focus should help to keep your mental powers in good order as you grow older.

improve your self-esteem

✔ Greater sense of pride in yourself.

✔ Improved self-confidence.

Regularly taking time to do something that makes you feel good enhances the rest of your life. You feel a sense of pride in your body every time it performs a movement that you previously thought would be impossible, such as touching your toes. The fact that you achieved this by connecting your mind and body gives you an amazing sense of empowerment. In addition, you become more accepting of your imperfections. What used to bug you about your body becomes one of the areas you're still working on and in which you expect to see results with continued practice.

The better you feel about yourself, the more you want to exercise and eat healthily. Feeling good about your body, whatever your size and shape, gives a new sense of self-assurance that attracts people to you. Self-confidence also happens to be the strongest aphrodisiac there is.

acquire a feeling of well-being

When you really concentrate on each exercise, you begin to understand what people mean when they talk about "being in the flow." You suddenly find yourself living fully in the present, not worrying about the future, nor feeling regretful about the past. The more this effect spills over into your daily life, the more able you are to *stay* in the moment. This fosters an innate sense of well-being. You become a better listener, you are more perceptive and more aware. You are more successful at work and in your relationships—you are happier. This sense of happiness stems from the quality of your movements in Pilates. At last you are in control of your body, and you are in tune with what you are doing.

Pilates can also improve your sex life, your circulation, and give you clearer, more radiant skin. Do you need any more reasons to start your program?

no such thing as a quick fix

Let's get real here. There is no such thing as a quick fix in any exercise regimen. Pilates will give you fabulous improvements in body and mind over time, but it is not going to give you supermodel or film-star looks overnight. Instead of searching for the impossible dream of perfection, aim to get the best body you possibly can. One that moves with grace and ease, one that looks strong, toned, flexible, and sexy. In thirty sessions you will start to see changes, but you need to continue with Pilates to see continued improvements.

Pilates will sculpt long, lean muscles. It will also increase your lean muscle mass, which means your body burns up calories faster, helping you to lose weight and keep it off, if that's what your body needs. Many people find they go down a clothing size without changing their eating habits.

If you are overweight and want to speed up weight loss, you should combine Pilates with a healthy diet and some cardiovascular exercise, to help reduce your body fat. Pilates can give you a cardiovascular workout at its more advanced level, but beginners will need to supplement their classes in the beginning.

Cardiovascular exercise need only be moderate. You will achieve results from a 30- to 60-minute session, three to five times per week, of brisk walking, swimming, or any other activity that raises the heart rate. You could do this after your Pilates routine three times per week, or exercise every day and alternate a Pilates class one day with cardio the next.

Forget crash diets, be honest with yourself—you know they don't work. As soon as you go back to your normal way of eating, the weight piles back on. Read books on healthy eating or visit a nutritionist and start to eat well. That usually means increasing fruit and vegetables in your diet, eating lean meat/fish/soya, and smaller portions of complex carbohydrates. You'll also need to cut down on processed foods, saturated fats, and sugars, but there's no harm in giving yourself the odd treat every once in a while to keep you going. Do all that and the weight will almost certainly come off.

get the balance right

Quite simply, if the energy going in is less than the energy expended, you'll lose weight. If it doesn't, you'll either need to eat a little less or exercise a little more. It isn't easy, and it's certainly not the way we would choose to eat if all foods were equal, but if we want to lose weight and keep it off, sadly that's the bottom line. Whatever you decide to do, try to find a healthy way of eating that honestly suits your lifestyle and includes foods that you actually like. It may sound daft, but you'll be amazed at how many people don't take either of these factors into account and wonder why they fail. Choosing something you can stick to is the best way of ensuring success.

The best rate of weight loss is 1–2 lbs (0.5–1 kg) a week, as this means you'll lose body fat rather than lean muscle and are more likely to keep the weight off. If you lose weight at that rate while taking your thirty Pilates classes spread over 10 weeks, you could safely lose up to 20 lbs (10 kg) by your thirtieth session.

Pilates principles

In Pilates, quality of movement is emphasized over mindless repetition, and this is achieved by following six fundamental principles: breathing, concentration, control, centering, precision, and flow. Remember that it takes time to improve body awareness and to lengthen and strengthen muscles, so be patient. Keep referring back to these principles, and, in time, you'll feel them within your body as you move.

breathing

Breathing is essential to life, so breathing well is vital. Many of us shallow-breathe, or don't fully expel the air from our lungs, so we almost never get a good breath of fresh air. Breathing better will:

✓ Improve your circulation.

✓ Rid your body of toxins.

✓ Improve your skin tone.

✓ Encourage concentration and help you to recruit the appropriate muscles for your movements.

✓ Calm your body and mind.

✓ Help you control your movements in daily life.

concentration

This is the key to connecting mind and body. It's the mind that makes the body move. Concentrate on each part of every exercise: the rhythm of your breath, the position of your head, the curve of your back, the bend in your legs, the straightness of your arms, etc. Pay attention to the individual muscles you are working and they will fire up with extra strength. As your concentration improves, you'll gain a heightened sense of body awareness so that you can recognize body sensation far more accurately. This new skill is essential for improving your Pilates technique and it's great for enhancing your sex life, too.

control

One of the most vital elements of Pilates is controlling your movements properly—Joseph Pilates originally called his new exercise program "Contrology." It is better to perform two exercise repetitions correctly, than twenty incorrectly. Badly performed exercises are the primary cause of injuries in other exercise methods. By carefully controlling your muscles, Pilates becomes one of the safest exercise programs around. Control is also required to ensure you get the maximum benefit from each exercise. Each detail of every movement serves a function.

centering

Think about the way you move: which muscles do you use most frequently? Most probably the muscles of your arms and legs. But there is a large group of muscles in the center of your body—starting from the pelvic floor muscles and including the muscles in the buttocks, hips, stomach, and back, all the way up to the lower ribs—which we all too often neglect. Joseph Pilates called this center the powerhouse (see page 18), and it is your powerhouse that you need to strengthen and use to support your spine, your internal organs, and your posture. Strengthening your powerhouse can reduce or eliminate many of the problems associated with chronic pain, and lower back pain in particular. It will also help your internal organs to function correctly and allow your limbs to move safely and gracefully around this strong core. Pilates teaches you how to initiate all of your movements from your center so that you function at your best, not just during your exercise routine but in your daily life. Centering in Pilates will also make you feel more stable, more secure, more able to rely upon yourself and worry less about others, which in turn boosts your confidence. It will affect your mental clarity and create a sense of deep tranquility.

precision

If you want to improve the quality of your movements, you need to use absolute precision. By thinking precisely, you can control specific muscles in your body. This allows you to move precisely so that you can realign or resculpt those muscles. Every exercise given in Pilates is there for a purpose, and every little instruction needs to be acted upon to ensure success. You should aim to practice to perform each movement perfectly; one perfect movement is better than several half-hearted ones. Eventually, that precision will become second nature.

flow

One of the most enjoyable things about Pilates is the freedom and grace you feel as you perform it. You're in the moment, what is sometimes called "being in the flow." None of the movements in Pilates are quick or jerky and there are no static, isolated movements because the body doesn't naturally move this way. Instead, grace triumphs over speed. There's the same fluidity you might feel if you were performing ballet or martial arts.

During your workout, try to concentrate on flow in each individual exercise. As you grow more practiced, flow as you move from one exercise to the next.

incorporating the principles

When you practice Pilates, try to keep the six fundamental principles in mind. You are learning to master your body with your mind, so just tackle one principle at a time before adding the next and soon it will become habitual:

First learn the steps and then the **breathing**.

Next **concentrate** on your body.

Move with **control**.

Initiate movements from your **center**.

Work with **precision**. Then establish a **flow**.

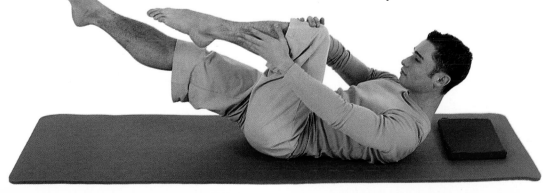

postural assessment

Before you begin your Pilates program, you need to take a closer look at your current posture so that you can fully appreciate the wonderful changes that await you.

how pilates can help

Stand as you normally would in front of a full-length mirror and study yourself from all angles—front, back, and sides. Better still, ask a friend or partner to take photographs of you in your underwear from these angles. Then have a look at the questions below—if you answer yes to any of them, Pilates should be able to help. It's not an overnight miracle, but slowly and steadily your posture can improve. Your first thirty Pilates classes are going to set you on your way. When your body is out of good alignment, it can cause problems: lower backaches, chronic neck and shoulder pain, weak knees, decreased lung capacity, compressed nerves, and frequent headaches, to name a few. Poor posture can also project underconfidence and feebleness.

Good posture, on the other hand, reduces aches and pains and means you move more gracefully and with greater ease. Your lungs can function more effectively, increasing your circulation and giving you more energy. Good posture implies confidence, vitality, and good health. In addition to your Pilates sessions, train yourself to improve your posture every day. Think of your alignment, whether you are standing, lying down, or sitting. Standing in good posture may seem strange at first as you're not used to it, but it will come with practice. By simply improving your posture, you will probably already "grow" an inch and reduce your waistline.

There are all kinds of different posture resulting from bad habits, genetics, or even disease. A good Pilates teacher will be able to diagnose your posture problems and recommend particular exercises to improve them. If you are generally fit, with no major problems, all of the Pilates exercises in this book will bring major postural benefits.

could you improve your posture?

● Instead of standing tall, are you slumping, adding inches to your waistline and reducing inches from your height?

● Does your head push forward in front of the rest of your body?

● Do your shoulders round forward putting your spine out of line?

● Is one shoulder higher than the other?

● Do you tense up both shoulders toward your ears, weakening your upper back muscles?

● Are you sticking your ribs and chest out, making your shoulders fall back?

● Do you have a potbelly, causing your lower back to arch excessively and possibly to ache?

● Do your knees and ankles roll inward or outward? Are your hips out of line with your knees, and your knees out of line with your ankles?

● Are your feet turning outward, giving you a faint resemblance to a duck?

standing in good posture

• Stand with your feet hip-width apart, making sure that your feet are facing forward, parallel to one another.

• Balance the weight evenly between the ball of your big toe, the outside edge of your foot, and the heel.

• Make sure both legs are facing forward.

• Keep your knees in a soft, unlocked position.

• Gently draw in your abdominal muscles and let your tailbone (coccyx) drop down. Imagine a tail made of lead attached to your tailbone, and feel it sink toward the floor between your legs.

• Stand up tall, so that there is plenty of space between your hips and your ribcage, making sure the ribs don't poke out.

• Unround your shoulders by gently lifting them up toward your ears and then circling them back and letting them drop down again. Keep them down by gently pressing your armpits toward your hips.

• Relax your arms so that they fall over the middle of your hips. Palms should face your sides and not face backward behind you.

• Lengthen the back of your neck. Imagine there is a rope attached to the crown of your head and it is being very gently drawn up toward the ceiling.

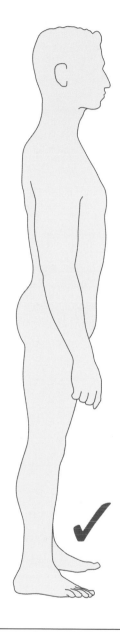

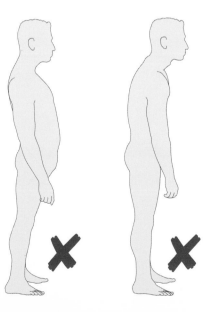

caution

If you have any kind of muscular-skeletal problem resulting from an injury or medical condition, such as slipped discs, osteoporosis, arthritis, or repetitive strain injury, it is essential that you discuss taking up this program with a doctor and a Pilates teacher before you do so. Pilates is almost certainly an excellent form of exercise for you to take up, but it should only be done under medical supervision.

anatomy

It is useful to be familiar with the structure of your skeleton and your basic muscle groups so that you can become more aware of how your body is moving when you practice Pilates. The following diagrams are by no means complete, but provide an handy overview of your musculoskeletal structure.

skeletal structure

1 Cervical vertebrae this upper section of the spine, the top seven vertebrae, is very flexible, allowing the head a wide range of movement. However, this flexibility makes the cervical spine particularly vulnerable to injury.

2 Thoracic vertebrae these twelve vertebrae articulate with the twelve pairs of ribs.

3 Lumbar vertebrae the five vertebrae between the ribs and the pelvis, which bear the weight of the whole torso.

4 Sacral vertebrae these five vertebrae are fused together in an adult to form solid bone.

5 Coccyx the bottom four vertebrae of the spine. They are fused together to form what is popularly known as the "tailbone."

6 Sternum this links with the top ten pairs of ribs, leaving the two lowest pairs floating.

7 Ribs these form a protective cage that shields some of the body's internal organs from injury (for example, the heart and lungs).

8 Pelvis made up of three fused bones, the wing-shaped ilium, the pubis in front, and the ischium behind. As a rough guide, if you imagine the triangle formed between your two hip bones and your pubic bone, and imagine a corresponding triangle at the back of your body, your pelvis lies between these two triangles.

9 Hip joint the ball-and-socket construction that connects the femur and pelvis.

10 Femur the thigh bone.

11 Fibula and Tibia the two bones of the lower leg.

12 Humerus the upper arm bone.

13 Radius and Ulna the lower arm bones.

muscles

1 Trapezius runs down the back of the neck and along the shoulders. *Used* to move the head, neck, and shoulder blades. The lower half, with the serratus anterior, rhomboid, and the latissimus dorsi muscles, is important for shoulder stability.

2 Deltoid encloses the shoulder and upper arm. *Used* for forward and backward movement, and for lifting the arm.

3 Rhomboid attaches the shoulder blade to the spine. Most of it lies beneath the trapezius muscle.

4 Triceps muscle of the upper arm. *Used* to straighten the arm.

5 Latissimus dorsi runs from the mid-thoracic to the lumbar region. *Used* to pull the shoulders down and back and the body upward.

6 Serratus anterior draws the shoulder blade forward against the ribs.

7 Erector spinae (not shown) group of muscles running along either side of the spine.

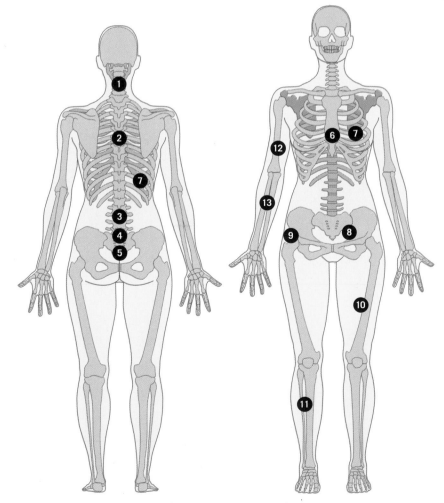

Used to keep the spine upright. The deep multifidus in the lumbo-sacral region plays a vital role in maintaining core stability along with the abdominal muscles.

8 Quadratus lumborum (not shown) or "lower back" muscle, a deep muscle at the side of the waist. **Used** primarily for side-bending.

9 Gluteus maximus forms the greater part of the buttock muscles. **Used** for running, jumping, and climbing.

10 Hamstrings three muscles that run down the back of the thigh.

Used to lift the thigh backward away from the body and to bend the leg at the knee.

11 Gastrocnemius forms the greater part of the calf muscles, and runs down the back of the lower leg. **Used** for flexing the foot.

12 Pectorals these chest muscles bring the arm toward the body. **Used** to rotate the arm, and flex and stabilize the shoulder.

13 Biceps muscle of the upper arm. **Used** to bend the elbow.

14 Rectus abdominis or "six pack"

muscles, run down the front of the abdomen. **Used** to bend the trunk, pulling the lower body toward the ribcage. Help to maintain good posture, working together with the deeper transversus abdominis (not shown) and the obliques.

15 External obliques abdominal muscles running diagonally along the sides of the trunk. **Used** to bend and rotate the trunk, working with the deeper internal obliques (not shown) and the rectus abdominis. Important for core stability.

16 Psoas (not shown) or "hip flexor." Two deep muscles running from the front of the femur, through the pelvis, to the lumbar region of the spine. **Used** to flex the thigh. Important for good pelvic stability.

17 Adductors four inner thigh muscles. **Used** for moving the leg inward.

18 Quadriceps or "quads." The quadriceps femoris is one muscle with four heads and runs down the front of the thigh. **Used** to perform the opposite movement to the hamstrings, extending or straightening the knee. It also acts on the hip joint to raise the thigh toward the hip.

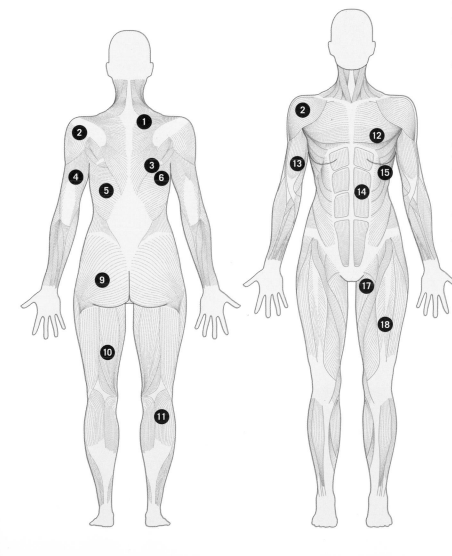

core stabilization

Core stabilization is the key to Pilates. You need to strengthen your trunk, your "center," in order to move most efficiently. If your center is strong, you are better balanced and this will have a dramatic impact on the rest of the body.

In core stabilization exercises, you create a "girdle of strength," the powerhouse, around your trunk to protect your spine and your internal organs. This can then be called upon to control your limbs while protecting your spine.

Many of us exercise without thinking about the beginning of each movement. As a result, we move poorly, which puts us at risk of straining our muscles or giving ourselves an even greater injury. Pilates will train you to recruit your powerhouse at the beginning of each movement. In each exercise, you start by strengthening your center before working any of the other muscles. In this way, you learn to initiate from the center of your body. This powerful technique will:

✓ Improve your alignment and posture.

✓ Radically reduce back pain.

✓ Strengthen and protect your body for life.

the powerhouse muscles

Joseph Pilates originally described this region as lying between the base of the ribs and the top of the pelvis, but nowadays the powerhouse refers to the area from the lower ribcage to the pelvic floor. Your abdominal muscles surround and support your lower torso and connect your pelvis to your ribs. The most important abdominal muscles (see diagram, right) form a corset that stabilizes your spine, protects your internal organs, and enables you to bend and twist.

The **rectus abdominis** is the easiest abdominal muscle to activate, but it needs to be controlled by the deeper abdominal muscles, the **transversus abdominis** and the **internal** and **external obliques**. These are usually the weakest and can often be forgotten when doing stomach crunches in the gym. For this reason, in Pilates you will work from the inside out, starting with the deeper layers of muscle and moving outward toward the more superficial muscle. You can only activate the deeper muscles by breathing well and that's why breathing plays such an important part in Pilates. Strengthening all your abdominal muscles, and not just the rectus abdominis, will make all the difference to achieving that firmer, flatter stomach.

Other muscles also play a key role in core stabilization. These include the muscles of your back, buttocks, your hip flexors, and even your pelvic floor. They work in conjuction with the abdominal muscles to stabilize your core. Pilates will strengthen every one of them and teach you to use them correctly when you move.

the abdominal muscles

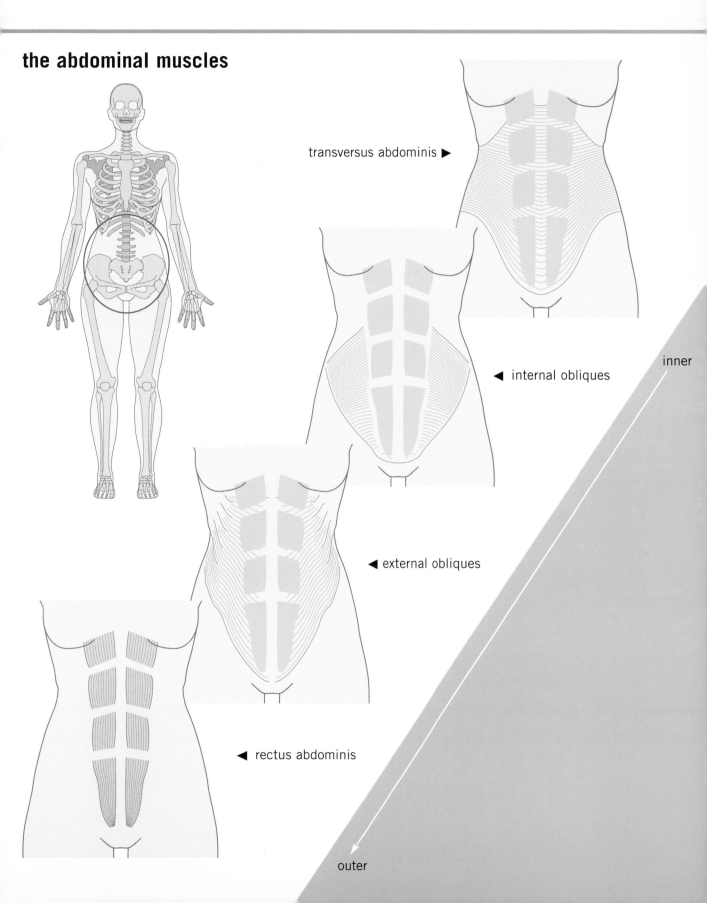

transversus abdominis ▶

internal obliques ▶

external obliques ▶

rectus abdominis ▶

inner

outer

shoulder stabilization

It is very common to overuse your deep supporting shoulder muscles or use them incorrectly, and this frequently leads to stiff, painful shoulders, plus chronic neck pain and headaches. Good shoulder stabilization will help to reduce these problems.

how to stabilize your shoulders

Holding your shoulder blades stable when you move allows your arms to reach or lift freely. Throughout this book, you'll be instructed to stabilize your shoulders, or slide your shoulder blades down into your back. To do this, think of drawing down the outsides of your shoulder blades so that they move downward toward your hips, or imagine you are sliding your armpits down toward your hips. Don't let the shoulder blades retract together as you perform the movement. They must not protrude or "wing." Instead, as you slide them down, think of them wrapping forward slightly toward the side of the ribcage. It's a small but vital movement.

As you exercise, if a movement is tricky to perform, you may find your shoulders are the first area to tense up. Rather than allowing this to happen, you need consciously to relax your shoulders during all the movements, by sliding the shoulder blade down your back.

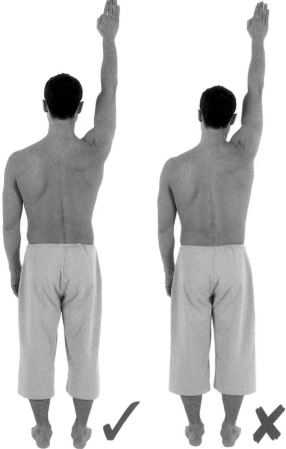

1 Stand in front of a mirror and slowly extend one arm forward and up to the ceiling. Now slowly take that straight arm down.

2 Examine that movement. When you lifted the arm above your head, was there space between the top of the shoulder and your ear? (See above left.) Or did your shoulder move up toward your ear, creating tension? (See above right.)

3 Try raising your arm again and this time focus on sliding the outside edge of the shoulder blade gently down and then lift your arm. This gives more space between the top of the shoulder and the ear and creates no tension. If you can only move your shoulder and arm up together, the joint is not working as it should. Pilates should help to free it up.

pelvic floor

The pelvic floor muscles are a sling of muscles in the pelvic area that support the internal organs and connect to the rest of the abdominal region. They are extremely important as they are fundamental to core stability and also interact with the thoracic region (the part of the body enclosed by the ribs), affecting your ability to breathe.

The pelvic floor is just like any other muscle. If you don't exercise it, it grows weak and can lead to problems. If your pelvic floor loses tone and elasticity, your posture collapses, your stomach protrudes, and the muscles that control your rectum, bladder, and your vagina, if you are a woman, weaken. A weak pelvic floor can lead to back pain and also incontinence (most often experienced by women after childbirth).

Since the outer muscles of the pelvic floor surround the sexual organs, strong pelvic floor muscles can also help sustain your libido. Improve your pelvic floor muscles, and you could also improve your sex life!

It helps to incorporate the pelvic floor in lateral breathing (see page 23).

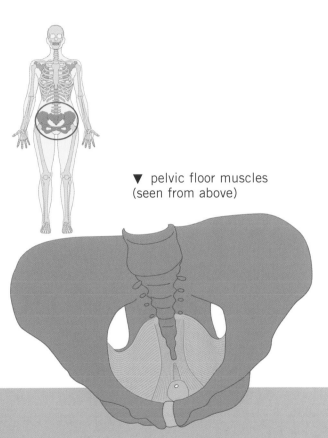

▼ pelvic floor muscles (seen from above)

how to find your pelvic floor

The easiest way for both men and women to find their pelvic floor is to stop the flow of urine briefly while urinating. The pelvic floor is the muscle you'll feel when you stop the flow. Try this a couple of times, just so you can locate it, but not on a regular basis as frequently stopping urine flow may not be good for your bladder in the long term.

• Learn to engage your pelvic floor muscles when you are standing, sitting, or lying down.

• Practice gently engaging and releasing your pelvic floor muscles regularly so that you can locate them easily. Women usually find it easiest to locate them if they imagine sucking water up into their vaginas.

Men are lifting their urethas and need only remember the feeling they get when they walk into icy-cold seawater. Recreating that "lift" works the pelvic floor muscle. Remember not to engage your buttock muscles as you lift.

breathing

If we breathe poorly, our lungs don't take in enough fresh oxygen for optimum health,

the ribcage region can become stiff and inflexible, and this can lead to back problems.

If we breathe well, we oxygenate the blood, dispel toxins, and circulation improves.

There are different ways of breathing badly. Some people are upper-chest breathers and take short shallow breaths, tightening the neck and the throat, lifting the shoulders and ribs with each inhalation. This is particularly stressful on the body and is very common among asthma sufferers. Others tend to be more diaphragmatic breathers, only filling out their stomachs with each breath.

lateral breathing

In Pilates, we practice what is known as lateral breathing as this provides greater **core stability**. By breathing more laterally, we expand our ribcage sideways with each breath, breathing air into the sides and back of the ribcage. This works the muscles between the ribs, facilitating their expansion, making the upper body more flexible.

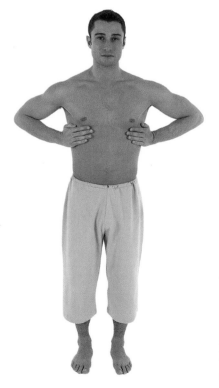

1 Place your hands on either side of your ribcage. **Breathe in slowly and gently** through your nose, allowing your ribs to expand outward laterally into your hands, as you try to fill the sides and back of your ribcage with air. Don't force the movement, your ribcage may only move slightly at first.

2 **Exhale slowly** through the mouth keeping your lips and jaw relaxed so that the lips are not pursed together and the jaw is not clenched.

3 Take 6–10 breaths in this manner.

4 Repeat 6–10 breaths but this time just allow your arms to rest by your sides.

It can take a while for lateral breathing to come naturally, particularly if your upper and mid-back are tight. Just keep practicing and it will eventually become second nature.

important note

The style of breathing described in this book is the basic way of Pilates breathing. It has been kept deliberately simple since you are learning at home without the benefit of supervised instruction. If you feel you have fallen into bad breathing habits and can't seem to get the hang of lateral breathing even after practicing diligently, it would be well worth taking a private lesson with a Pilates instructor who would be able to teach you better breathing.

drawing in the abdominals

When we breathe laterally in Pilates, we also incorporate the abdominal muscles and pelvic floor in our movements for even greater core stability.

Breathing this way will feel very different to start with, but keep practicing the method described below. To begin with, you may find you inhale into your upper chest or your stomach as well as into your ribcage. That's fine for now—if your ribcage is stiff and inflexible, it may take a while before it begins to move more freely. Try lateral breathing and drawing in the abdominals while sitting and standing, as well as while lying down. This will strengthen your deep abdominal muscles, which have probably been underused. These are the muscles that will help to give you a flat stomach and protect you from lower back pain.

If you are finding it difficult to locate your pelvic floor muscles, or can't seem to be able to engage them smoothly and gently without tightening your buttock muscles, then just leave the pelvic floor out for the moment and focus on drawing in the abdominals correctly on each exhalation. You can always go back to incorporating the pelvic floor when you become more experienced.

1 Lie on your back, with your knees bent at a 90-degree angle, and your feet and knees hip-width apart. Rest your arms by your sides. **Inhale** gently through the nose, taking the breath in laterally, filling the sides and back of your ribcage with air. Pause momentarily.

2 As you start to **exhale slowly** through the mouth, gently engage your pelvic floor, and as you **exhale**, feel your lower stomach start to sink down toward the floor. As you **continue to exhale**, allow your stomach to sink down a little further by drawing in your lower stomach muscles. Your stomach will hollow out. Don't brace your stomach muscles, just sink them gently downward and make sure you don't move your spine. Pause momentarily.

3 Gently **inhale** through your nose into the sides and back of your ribcage. Pause momentarily, then repeat the exhalation as above.

Repeat for 6–10 full breaths.

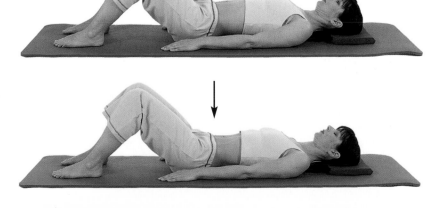

neutral spine

Most of the exercises in this book are performed in what is known as "neutral spine"

position. This describes the natural curves of your back and is usually the best position

for your spine, as it places the least stress on the spine and therefore protects the back.

finding your neutral spine

Neutral spine allows the best alignment of the body so that the muscles are well balanced. It also ensures you are engaging your abdominal muscles correctly. It is unique to the individual, so finding the position that is right for you may take a little practice.

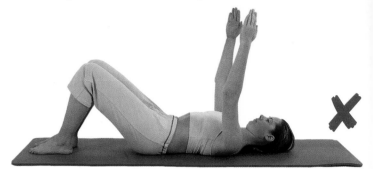

✘ Lie down on the floor with your knees bent. If you tilt your pelvis up (by rocking your pubic bone up toward the ceiling), you will lose the natural curve in your back as your spine flattens into the floor and your tailbone lifts off it.

✘ If you tilt your pelvis the other way (by rocking your pubic bone down to the floor), your back overarches.

✔ The neutral spine position lies between these two positions. Your pelvis is balanced so that the curve in your lower spine behind your waist is not completely lost by pressing your back into the floor, nor is your back overarched leaving a big gap between your back and the floor.

When you are in neutral, your tailbone (coccyx) remains on the floor and lengthens away, and your pubic bone and two hipbones are level with each other. Everyone's position will be slightly different, but in most cases there should be just

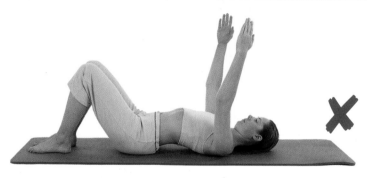

enough room for someone to slide a flat hand in the slight gap behind your waist when you are in neutral spine.

In Pilates, you want to work in neutral spine when you are standing, sitting, or lying down with your feet on the floor. If your feet are lifted off the mat, then you can come out of neutral and allow your lower back to press into the floor for additional support.

spinal articulation

Your spine is made up of 24 small bones (vertebrae) plus your sacrum and coccyx bones. The bones of the spine support your torso and protect your spinal cord. They also allow you to move. A flexible spine lets you twist, turn, and spiral in many different directions.

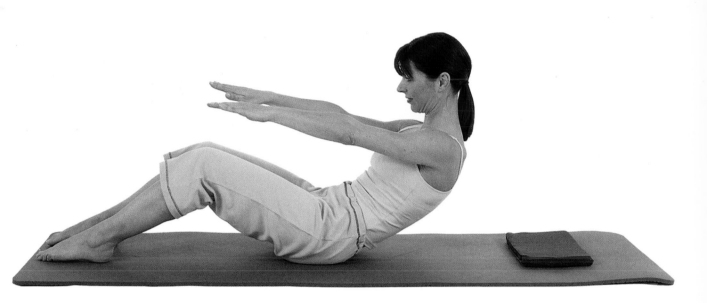

To create a flexible spine, you need to stretch and articulate it. You also need to strengthen it to improve your posture. Many Pilates exercises work on strengthening and increasing flexibility in the spine. In many of them you will read expressions such as "roll down the spine," "curl up the spine," or "peel the spine off the mat one vertebra at a time." All this really means is articulating your spine so that you work through each section of the spine, mobilizing and separating each vertebra so they move one at a time.

As you curl up and down your spine, you will be aware that some sections feel flexible, while others feel stiff and tight, and hard to separate from each other. These tight areas are the areas you must really focus on, taking your time, and breathing slowly to increase the opening of the area. Whether you are rolling up or down, imagine you are curving your spine into the shape of a letter C each time you move, as this will help you to articulate better through the spine thus increasing flexibility and strength.

alignment

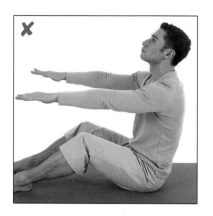

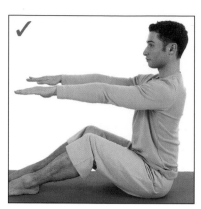

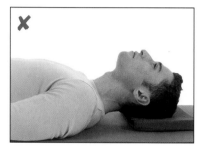

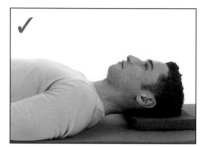

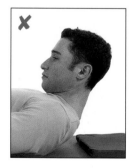

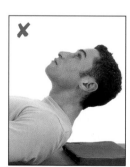

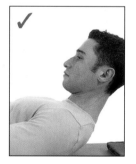

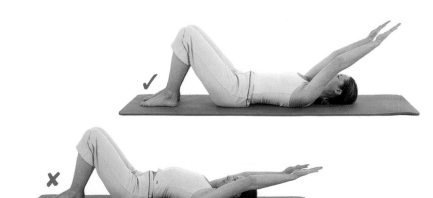

head position

Crunching the vertebra at the back of your neck can lead to neck and shoulder tension, pain, and poor posture. When **sitting** or **standing**, think of lengthening through the crown of your head to elongate the back of your neck. *Imagine a piece of rope attached to your crown being gently drawn up to the ceiling.*

When **lying** on your back, use a head rest for support and gently elongate the back of your neck. Lower your chin slightly toward your chest, but still leave a gap the size of a peach between your chin and chest.

If your head and shoulders are **lifted** off the mat, lengthen through the crown of the head to elongate the back of your neck. Your head should be above your breastbone with a peach-sized gap between chin and chest. Your abdominal muscles and the back of your chest support you so you don't strain the neck muscles.

ribcage

Sticking the ribs out and up when raising the arms will cause you to arch your lower back and strain your neck and shoulders. If you notice your ribs "popping out," correct this by gently sliding your ribcage down the front of your body toward your hips. This lengthens your spine and stops your back from arching.

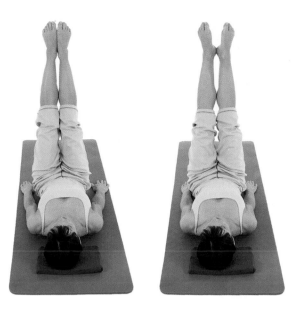

turning the legs out

Occasionally, you'll be asked to turn your legs out. This position involves rotating your thighs outward in the hip sockets so that your heels come together, and very gently engaging the lower part of your buttocks as if you were holding a coin between them. If you do this correctly, you will also feel the muscles at the top of your inner thighs engage. If you are lying down, try not to lift your tailbone as you engage but lengthen your legs away from you to keep your leg muscles stretched. Working in this turned out position ensures that you work the correct muscles to tone up your hips, buttocks, and thighs and stabilize your lower body.

working in opposition

Muscles tend to work in pairs or groups. For example, if you lift one arm up and bend it at the elbow, your bicep muscle at the front of your upper arm is working to make the bending movement. For the movement to happen, however, the muscle at the back of your upper arm (the tricep) has to lengthen to allow the bicep to bend.

Other muscles in your body also have to work when you bend your arm to stop your whole body from bending over with it. These are called stabilizer muscles. If one muscle reaches away from your body, at least one other also has to work to keep your body counterbalanced so that you don't tip over. As you practice Pilates, you will need to train yourself to emphasize these opposing movements.

body alignment

When you are performing the exercises, it is essential that you do them symmetrically so that your body develops symmetrically. Imagine a square in the center of your body that runs from shoulder to shoulder, shoulder to hip, hip to hip, and shoulder to hip. Try to keep this square shape, or "box" as it is sometimes called, as you perform the exercises.

People often favor one side of the body more than the other and being aware of this will keep you in alignment, so that you don't lean over too far to one side, or twist too far to the other as you exercise.

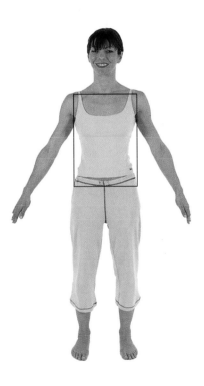

preparation week

Don't be in a hurry to advance into your Pilates program. The best way to begin is to lay the foundations first. Read the Introduction a few times and practice the basics (see opposite). Don't worry if it doesn't all make complete sense immediately. As you begin to practice Pilates, it will all start to fall into place.

Ideally, one week before you start your Pilates program, try lateral breathing (see page 22) and drawing in the abdominal muscles (see page 23). Try 10 full breath cycles (breathing in and out is one full cycle) three times per day. Breathing like this for a week before you begin your program will begin to strengthen those deep abdominal muscles that are so important for your posture. If you can begin to do this before you start, you'll find you progress far more quickly.

what you need

the space

Choose a warm, quiet space where you like to be and that you can make your own three times a week. If you can keep your mat out all the time, so that you're already set up, so much the better. You may wish to add candles and flowers, and play some quiet relaxing music. Make the space as much of a sanctuary as you can, so that you'll want to come in and practice. If you can only find space by clearing away the kids' toys in front of the sofa, that's fine. Make the area as comfortable as it can be, and then just start.

the mat

Use a mat to protect your spine. A Pilates mat is ideal, but you can use a yoga mat, which is slightly thinner. You can purchase either at most sports shops. If a mat is not available, use blankets or towels to create a cushioned surface on which you can lie full-length. A surface that is too soft is not good as it may inhibit balance and make it hard to control your movements.

the head rest

For all the exercises performed lying down, it is useful to use a head rest. This will support the head, and help to lengthen the neck, relax the shoulders, and facilitate better breathing. Either use a book, about an inch thick and large enough to place your head on without it rolling off, or make your own head rest by using an inch-thick cut of foam. When you are more experienced, you may no longer need a head rest, but it is very helpful for your first 30 Pilates sessions.

frequency

Practice your routine three times per week, ideally leaving one day in between for the body to rest. Try to stick to a regular Monday/Wednesday/Friday or a regular Tuesday/Thursday/Sunday pattern, if you can. The more you can make it a routine, the more easily Pilates will become a habit for life. If you have to miss a day, just make sure you make up for it later in the week so, even if you end up having to practice two days in a row, you still complete your three sessions that week.

maintaining motivation

If it's your regular day to practice and you don't feel like it, try striking a deal with yourself: you just have to lie down on the mat and do one exercise. If, after that, you still don't feel like exercising, that's fine, you can leave it for that day. The chances are, the first exercise will start to feel so good that, before you know it, you'll want to continue.

basics to practice before you start

caution

● Leave at least one hour after eating before performing your Pilates program.

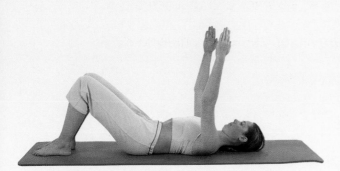

● **Find your neutral spine (see page 24).**

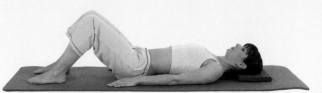

● **Find your pelvic floor (see page 21).**

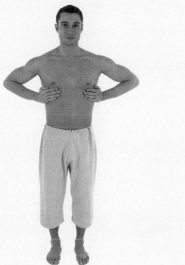

● **Practice lateral breathing (see page 22).**

● **Practice drawing in your abdominals (see page 23).**

● **Check out your shoulder stabilization (see page 20).**

● **Practice your standing posture (see page 15).**

● **Learn how to lengthen the back of your neck (see page 26).**

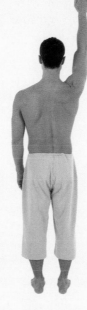

following the program

A full program of exercises takes you through your first thirty Pilates lessons and beyond. Everyone should start at Level 1 and work through all three levels, doing the exercises in the given order. Exercises range from beginners' to early intermediate and can be tailored to suit individual needs.

doing the exercises

Everyone's body is different and you will find some exercises challenge your own particular body structure more than others. That's fine. There is no competition and no rush. Go at your own pace, only progressing according to the instructions given when you are sure your body is ready to move on. When you first perform an exercise, stick to the low end of the range of repetitions given. Only when you are sure you have mastered it should you do the top number of recommended repetitions. Never do more than suggested. It's like doubling your medication to get better quicker; it won't give you better results!

transitions

At the end of each exercise, transition instructions are given to help you move smoothly from one exercise to the next. As you advance your routine, try to include these movements. Once you get practiced at it, your whole routine should become one seamless movement with no pauses in between. It flows and has a meditative quality to it.

modifications

These are suggested to help you decrease, or occasionally increase, the intensity of the movement to suit your needs. Always read the Modifications first to see if they apply to you before attempting the main, more traditional version.

Only give your body the level of exercise that it requires. To get results, you need to be able to perform the exercise correctly, following every little detail, and to feel challenged without feeling that you are straining in any way. The challenge may come from any aspect of the exercise—the muscle strength required to perform it, your flexibility, your alignment, your stability, or your endurance.

injuries

Caution Boxes are included beside the exercises for anyone with injuries. The exercises are suitable for adults of all ages who are generally fit and well and suffering from no injuries or medical conditions. The **Caution Box** is only a basic guideline and cannot possibly cover every eventuality. If you have an injury or medical condition or are in any doubt as to whether a particular exercise is appropriate for your body, consult a doctor and a qualified instructor.

Pilates can be great for all sorts of remedial work, and for certain medical conditions, but only under the supervision of your doctor and a qualified instructor. See a professional first, and then ask for guidance on which exercises in this book are suitable or unsuitable for you.

If you find an exercise is putting a strain on your body, stop, reread the instructions and check you are doing it correctly. Try again and if you still feel strain, and the suggested modification doesn't help, stop, and skip that exercise for now. As your strength and flexibility increase, try it again. Remember that some exercises may not be suitable for your body. Learn to listen to your body and only do what feels right for you.

listen to your body

Pilates should never be painful. An exercise may be hard work to perform, but it should never hurt, and you should never feel you are straining in any way.

backs

If you have no back injury or medical condition but feel a diffuse ache in your lower back while performing any of the exercises, this may be because you are not drawing in your abdominal muscles properly to protect your spine. Or it may be that your abdominal muscles are not yet strong enough to perform the movement. Try a modified version of the exercise, or reduce the number of repetitions until your abdominal muscles gain strength. If necessary, skip the exercise for the moment so you work without back tension. Exercises done when you are lying flat on your back, and therefore supported by the ground beneath you, are usually considered the safest ones for backs. **The exercises that are generally viewed as most challenging for bad backs are ones that involve rolling, arching, and twisting movements.**

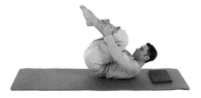

necks

If you have a weak neck, you should proceed with caution.

Remember to stay lifted using your abdominal muscles when performing a movement, and never lift with the neck itself. If your neck aches when lifting your head up while lying down, simply rest your head on your head rest for a while between repetitions, or perform the exercise with your head down. If it's more comfortable for you, exercise with a cushion or a rolled towel underneath your head to provide support until you grow stronger.

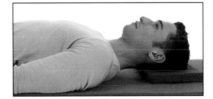

shoulders, elbows, and wrists

If you have weak wrists, elbows, or shoulders, you need to be extremely careful with weight-bearing exercises on your upper limbs. For shoulders and elbows, in particular, reduce the range of movement, working very slowly in a shortened range.

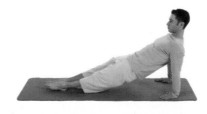

knees and ankles

If you have weak knees or ankles, you will need to be very careful with weight-bearing exercises on your lower limbs, such as those performed kneeling. You also need to avoid overextending your knees or bending them in too tightly as this might aggravate them. Knee pain can sometimes be caused by improper leg and foot positioning, so pay particular attention to your alignment. Try to maintain a "soft knee," bending it very slightly so it isn't locked while performing the movements.

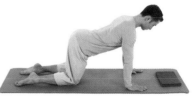

hips

If you feel a slight ache in the hip while moving one or both of your legs in the air, and have no injury or medical condition, try bending the knee slightly.

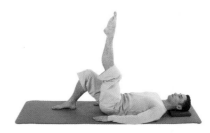

self-assessment

As you work through each exercise, you need to monitor each movement. It is the attention to detail in Pilates that will change your body and your life.

beginner's pelvic tilt

Before you start your Pilates program, try this exercise very slowly, then give yourself a body scan (see opposite).

If the exercise feels tough, or if you feel any tension in your back, shoulders, chest, or neck, don't come up so far from the floor. Just come up halfway until you grow stronger and more flexible.

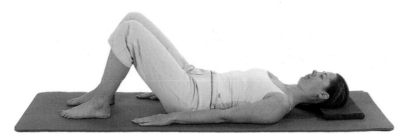

1 Lie on your back with your knees bent at a 90-degree angle, feet parallel and hip-width apart. Your arms reach long by your sides with your palms facing down. Place your head on your head rest and draw your chin down slightly to ensure that the back of your neck is long (see page 26). Breathe laterally (see page 22), **inhaling** slowly and gently through the nose.

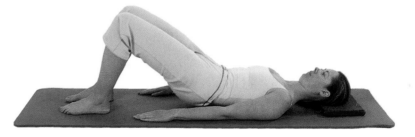

2 **Exhale**, engaging your pelvic floor and drawing in your abdominals (see page 23) as you peel your spine off the mat one vertebra at a time (see page 25) so that your hips curl up toward the ceiling. Press through your feet as you start to lift off, curling up as far as your body can go comfortably with the abdominals still engaged.

caution

● Proceed only under supervision if you have any back injuries or disc problems.

precision points

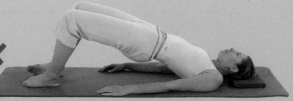

✗ Don't allow your knees to fall any further apart.

✗ Don't tense your neck, shoulders, and chest. Keep the back of your neck long.

body scan

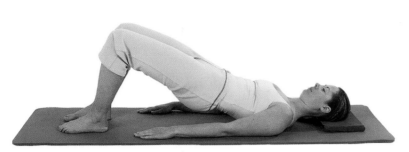

3 **Inhale**, holding your body perfectly still.

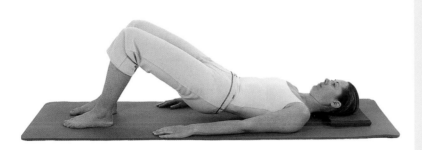

4 **Exhale**, engaging the pelvic floor and drawing in your abdominals, as you use them to roll down through your spine, lowering one vertebra at a time.

Imagine your spine is melting into the mat as you peel down.

how did it feel?

Did you find the exercise challenging? Did it take all your concentration? The answer to both questions should be yes if you performed the exercise correctly. Try it again, this time even more slowly and precisely. Now how did it feel? What felt challenging? Was it the movement? The breathing? Or the fact that there were so many details to think about?

✓ Try to isolate the vertebrae more each time you repeat the exercise.

✓ Relax the buttocks and be careful not to arch your lower back.

✓ Bring your tailbone down onto the mat last: take care not to lower your bottom to the floor before you have rolled through each vertebra in your lower back.

Try three more repetitions. As you are moving, ask yourself:

• Are my feet hip-width apart?

• Am I gently engaging my pelvic floor without clenching my buttocks?

• Am I drawing in my deep abdominal muscles continuously as I roll up and down?

• Am I breathing correctly?

• Are my shoulders stabilized?

• Can I feel my spine articulating one vertebra at a time?

• Am I including every detail of the exercise?

When you practice, aim initially to perform a movement safely and correctly, assessing yourself as you go. As your practice develops, keep referring back to the Precision Points to improve your style. Check the Poor Posture photograph to ensure you are not slipping into any bad habits. As your technique improves further, refer to the six Pilates Principles (see pages 12–13) and try to include them in your movements.

You won't manage to get it all right at first, but continue this self-assessment for each exercise, and soon you will be truly practicing Pilates. Learn how to monitor every last detail and then you can learn how to improve on them.

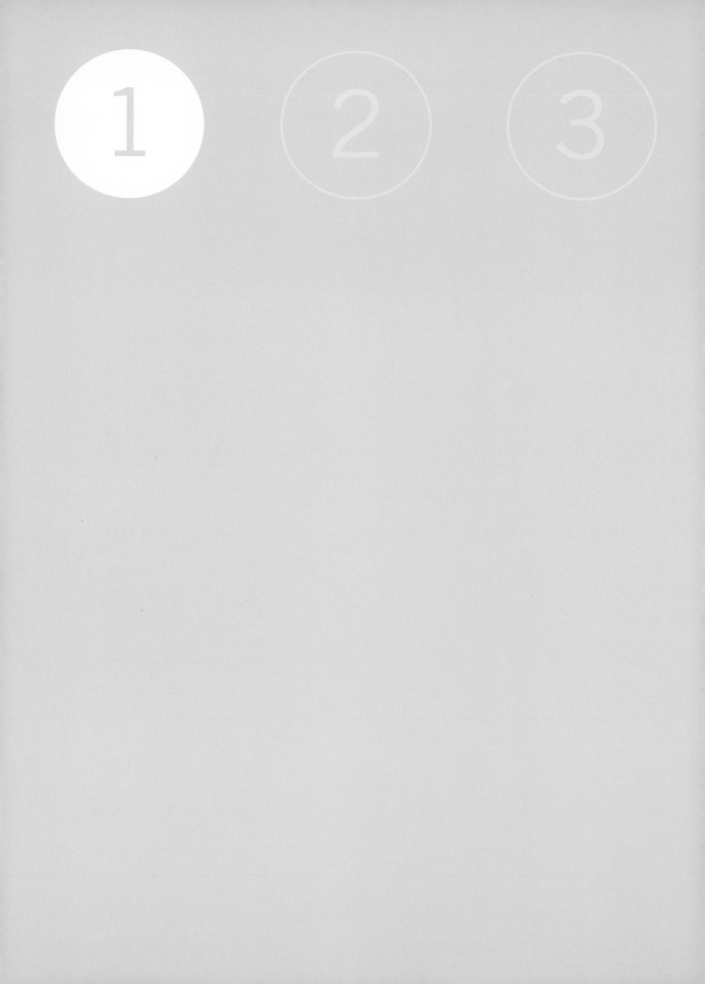

feel the difference

benefits after 10 sessions

Practice Pilates for just ten sessions and you will definitely feel the difference:

• You will probably feel better about yourself than you have in a long while.

• Your posture will improve—you'll be standing taller and your abdominal muscles will be held in better.

• You will breathe better, which will improve your circulation, your metabolism, and your skin tone.

• You will discover which parts of your body are weakest, and which parts need to become more flexible. Whichever part of your body needs most work, you will feel first.

• You will find your center, your core stability. Your abdominal muscles will start to firm up, even if you can't see it yet, and your pelvic floor muscles will strengthen. You will begin to initiate your movements from your powerhouse.

• You will also learn how to stabilize your shoulders and lengthen the back of your neck so that years of neck and shoulder tension can begin to ease, and your shoulder and arm movements can improve.

• As you lubricate your joints and stretch out your muscles, you will generally begin to feel less stiff. Stress can often make your flexibility worse because when you are stressed your muscles constrict and tighten around your joints. This can lead to back aches, neck and shoulder tension, headaches, and so on. One of the things you will be doing in your first ten classes is learning to lengthen these muscles away from the joint. After each Pilates session, you will feel your stress levels decrease and you will come away feeling relaxed and invigorated.

• The combination of increased flexibility and core stability means you will move with greater ease. Your movements will actually feel more fluid. Enjoy this new quality of movement. Feel good about it. It's bringing quality into your life that makes you feel good about yourself.

level 1 program

You should now have familiarized yourself with the contents of the Introduction and hopefully feel inspired to begin your Pilates exercises. Let's get started at Level 1.

Practice the Level 1 sequence of exercises three times per week, preferably exercising with one day's rest in between each session. Read all the instructions through first before attempting a movement, including the suggested modifications in case they apply to you. You need to make sure you give each exercise your full concentration. You want to feel the exercises are challenging you but never to the point of feeling strain. If in doubt, always select the easier modified version. Stick to the order of exercises given according to the **Exercise Sequence Chart** (see pages 38–39) and only skip one if you have an existing injury or medical condition that prevents you from performing the movement safely. Always look out for the caution boxes if you have any kind of injury, and if so, exercise only under supervision.

building the foundation

Level 1 is definitely the most important stage of learning Pilates. This is where you lay the foundations upon which you will build to achieve a strong and flexible body. Level 1 may seem easy but take your time. Don't breeze through it without paying attention. These exercises are your introduction to Pilates and are probably the most crucial part of the whole program. This is the time to start to put the theory of Pilates into practice. Your goal is to start to become aware of your body, to find the muscles you need for core stability and shoulder stability, to practice putting lateral breathing into action and to begin to strengthen your body, particularly your deep abdominal muscles for the more challenging exercises to come.

Remember to concentrate on what your body is feeling as you learn new movements and discover new muscles. When you're doing Level 1 exercises correctly, they are much harder than they first appear. Take your time to get the fundamentals right, and you'll really reap the benefits later. The Level 1 exercises introduce you to various muscle groups in your body. If you are doing them correctly, you should be able to isolate them while holding the rest of your body relaxed and still. To begin with you may feel you're not in control of your own body. For example, instead of doing a chest lift in a neutral spine position, you suddenly find you're out of neutral, your shoulders are lifting up toward your ears, and you are incorrectly thrusting your hips to the ceiling. Be patient and be precise. You'll soon replace these old postural habits with healthy new ones. You'll find teaching your body new tricks is a lot of fun.

when to progress to level 2

Move to Level 2 whenever you feel ready. If you are pretty fit, do the Level 1 exercises at least three times before moving on to Level 2 to ensure you have incorporated all the Pilates concepts mentioned in the Introduction. If you haven't exercised for a while and your muscles are weak or you feel very stiff, you may need to stay at Level 1 for ten or twenty sessions then decide for yourself. As long as you feel challenged and you're performing the exercises correctly, you'll get the benefits.

Continue to assess yourself as you perform the exercises (see Self-assessment, pages 32–33), and when you feel ready and able, move on to Level 2. Level 2 exercises still include many of the introductory exercises you learned in Level 1 but there are some additional exercises, all of which are much more challenging.

level 1: exercise sequence char

This Exercise Sequence Chart serves as a visual aid while you perform your program. When performed in the order shown, your movements will flow smoothly from one to the next. Position this book so you can see the chart easily from your mat. As you become more practiced, you will only need to refer to the chart to complete your routine.

1

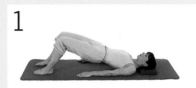

pelvic tilt p40

2

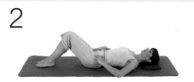

small hip roll p42

3

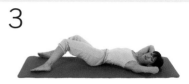

hip roll p44

7

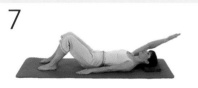

arm splits p52

8

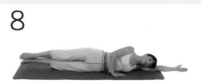

double leg lift p54

9

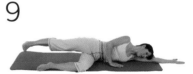

outer thigh lift p56

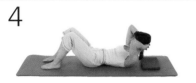

4 chest lift p46

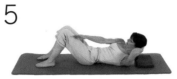

5 oblique reaches p48

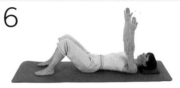

6 chest opener p50

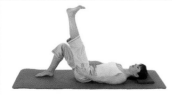

10 inner thigh lift p58

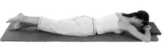

11 hamstring lift p60

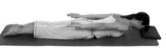

12 arrow (+ rest position) p62

stretches

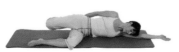

hamstring stretch p64

quadriceps stretch p65

buttock stretch p66

pelvic tilt

body benefits

- strengthens the abdominal muscles

- increases spinal flexibility

- mobilizes the shoulders

- relieves most minor backache and stiffness

repetitions: 6–10

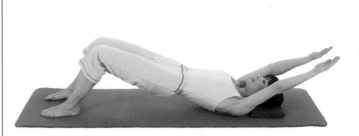

3 **Inhale**, holding your body perfectly still, and raise your arms up to the ceiling and then over toward your head until they are in line with your ears.

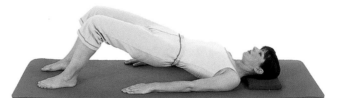

2 **Exhale**, drawing in your abdominals as you peel your spine off the mat one vertebra at a time so that your hips curl up toward the ceiling. Press through your feet as you start to lift off, curling up as far as your body can comfortably go with the abdominals still engaged.

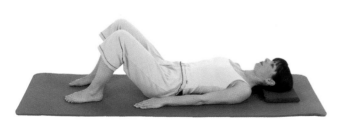

1 Lie on your back with your knees bent at a 90-degree angle, feet parallel to each other and hip-width apart. Arms reaching long by your sides with the palms facedown. Draw your chin down slightly to ensure that the back of your neck is long. **Inhale**.

precision points

✘ Don't allow your knees to fall any further apart.

✘ Don't tense the neck, shoulders, and chest. Keep back of neck long.

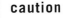

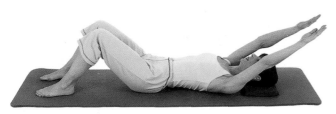

caution

● Proceed only under supervision if you have any back injuries or disc problems.

4 **Exhale**, drawing in the abdominals as you use them to roll down through your spine, lowering one vertebra at a time, leaving your arms behind you. *Imagine your spine softening and melting into the mat as you roll down.*

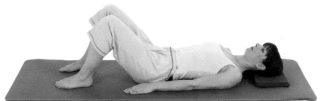

5 **Inhale**, lowering your arms to your sides. Repeat Steps 2–5 for required repetitions.

Transition: Bring your feet and knees together for the Small Hip Roll (see page 42), or lift your knees one at a time up toward your chest for the Side-to-Side (see page 74).

modifications

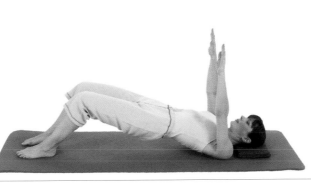

If the exercise feels tough, or if you feel any tension in your back, shoulders, chest, or neck, just come up halfway until you grow stronger and more flexible.

If you have shoulder problems, it may feel more comfortable to raise your arms to the ceiling rather than overhead, or just keep them on the floor. Keep the shoulder blades down into the back in both cases.

✓ **Try to isolate the vertebrae more each time you repeat the exercise.**

✓ **Bring your tailbone down onto the mat last: take care not to lower your bottom to the floor before you have rolled through each vertebra in your lower back.**

✓ **Relax the buttocks and be careful not to arch your lower back.**

small hip roll

body benefits

- strengthens and lengthens the abdominal muscles

- releases tension stored in the back and neck

- once the back and neck are freed up, posture immediately improves

repetitions: 10 each side, alternating sides

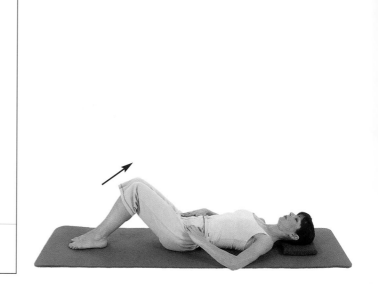

2 **Inhale**, rolling the knees to one side while pressing your opposite hand gently down on the hip to keep your hips and buttocks glued to the floor. You will not be able to go very far.

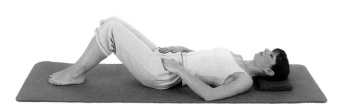

1 Lie on your back, with your knees bent at a 90-degree angle and feet together. Place your hands on your hips. Keep the back and the neck long.

precision points

✗ **Don't allow your knees to fall apart.**

✗ **Don't twist your body.**

1 2 3

caution

● This exercise is safe for most back injuries but always check with your doctor if you have any kind of back problem.

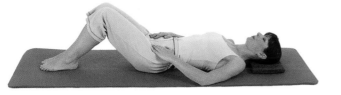

3 **Exhale**, drawing in the abdominals to return the knees to the center. *Imagine your thighs are made of lead so that you really have to use your abdominal muscles to swing your knees back to center each time.*

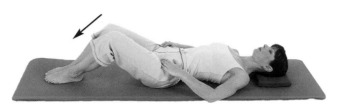

4 **Inhale** to take the knees over to the other side, while pressing gently down on the hip with the opposite hand.

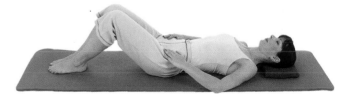

5 **Exhale**, drawing in the abdominals again to return the knees to the center.

Transition: Take the feet a little wider than hip-width apart for the Hip Roll (see page 44).

modifications

If your back is very stiff, don't take the knees as far over. Keep the movement very small at first.

✓**Be careful not to take your knees over too far, or your back, hips, and bottom will lift.**

✓**Keep your knees tightly together throughout.**

✓**Roll straight from side to side with no twisting.**

hip roll

body benefits

- strengthens the abdominal muscles

- stretches the hip flexors and lower back

- releases tension in the upper spine

- great for people with stiff shoulders, backs, or necks

- once upper body tension is reduced, breathing improves

repetitions: 10 each side, alternating sides

modifications

If you feel tension in your lower back, don't take your knees over so far. If it still feels uncomfortable, just stick to the Small Hip Roll (see page 42) until you become stronger and more flexible.

If placing your hands behind your head is uncomfortable, reach the arms long by your sides with the palms facing down instead.

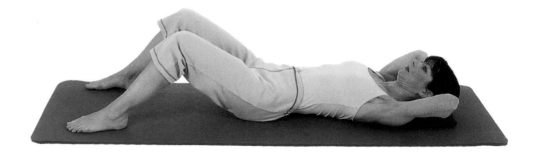

1 Lie on your back with your knees bent at a 90-degree angle and your feet slightly wider than hip-width apart. Your neck is long and your spine relaxed. Bend your arms and place both hands beneath your head, elbows wide. **Inhale**.

precision points

✗ Don't twist so far that your shoulder blades lift off the mat.

1 2 3

caution

● Omit this exercise if you have a bad neck or back injury.

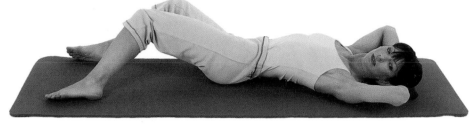

2 **Exhale**, drawing in the abdominals, as you roll your knees toward the floor. The soles of your feet will come off the mat. As you stretch, let your head roll in the opposite direction to your knees so that you feel a stretch through your body. **Inhale** and rest in this position.

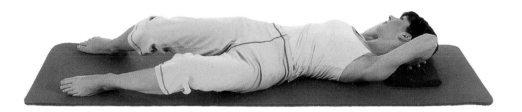

3 **Exhale**, drawing in the abdominals, to roll your knees all the way over to the other side. Let your head roll in the opposite direction. Imagine your lower abdominal muscles sinking down through your spine toward the floor. **Inhale** and rest in this position. Alternate smoothly from side to side.

Transition: Return to Step 1 position and move feet back to hip-width apart for the Chest Lift (see page 46).

✓ Make sure your shoulder blades stay glued to the mat throughout.

✓ Only move when you are exhaling. Remain still as you inhale.

✓ Try to think of relaxing the fronts of your thighs as you move, and use the hollowing of the abdominals to initiate swinging the knees from one side to the other.

chest lift

body benefits

- strengthens the abdominal muscles for a firmer, flatter stomach

- highlights shoulder stabilization and neutral spine position

repetitions: 6–10

modifications

If your abdominal muscles start to quiver or pop out as you roll up, don't come up so high for the moment.

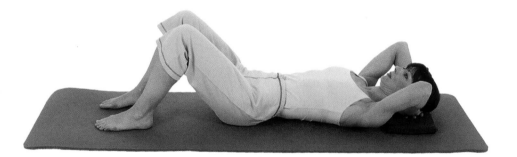

1 Lie on your back with your knees bent, feet and knees hip-width apart. Bend your arms to fold your hands behind your head, fingers interlaced and elbows out to the side. Check you are in neutral spine position. **Inhale**.

precision points

✗ Don't let your shoulder blades lift.

✗ Don't come out of your neutral spine position.

1 2 3

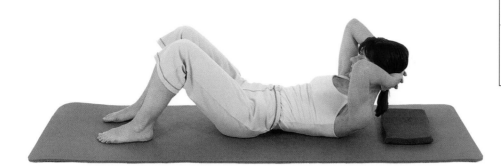

2 **Exhale**, drawing in the abdominals, to roll your head and shoulders off the mat. As you roll up, slide your shoulder blades down into your back to keep the tops of your shoulders away from your ears. Keep your chin toward your chest with only a small space in between. *Imagine you are gently holding a peach under your chin*. **Inhale** and remain perfectly still in this lifted position.

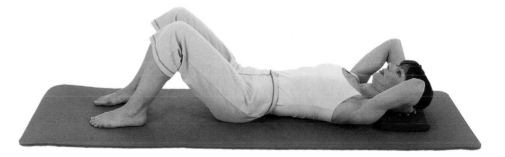

3 **Exhale**, drawing in the abdominals to roll your head and shoulders back on to the mat.

Transition: Leave one arm behind your head and cross your other arm over to your opposite hip bone for the Oblique Reaches (see page 48), or take both arms by your sides and lift your knees toward your chest, one leg at a time, to prepare for The Hundred (see page 106).

✓ Watch that the shoulder blades stay down into the back throughout to maintain good shoulder stabilization.

✓ Make sure your abdominal muscles keep drawing in so they don't pop out as you roll up. There should be no tension in the back.

✓ Support the weight of your head in your hands so there is no tension in the neck.

oblique reaches

body benefits

- strengthens the abdominal muscles (internal and external oblique muscles in particular, hence the name)

- trims the waist

repetitions: 6–10 each side

modifications

If you can't maintain neutral spine, and find you are tucking under and pressing your lower back into the mat, don't come up so high.

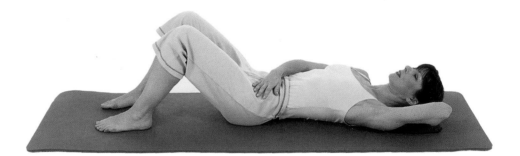

1 Lie on your back with your knees bent, feet hip-width apart. Bend one arm to fold one hand behind the head. The other hand rests on the opposite hipbone. **Inhale**.

precision points

✗ Don't let your tailbone lift off the floor to come out of neutral spine.

✗ Don't twist from your shoulders. Twist from your ribcage instead.

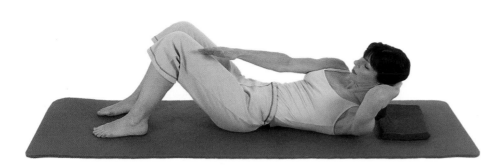

caution

● Proceed only under supervision if you have a neck or back injury.

2 **Exhale**, drawing in the abdominals to cross your arm over your body, stretching diagonally toward the outside of your opposite knee. Your palm faces down. Stay in neutral position, rotating your lower ribcage over to the side rather than just twisting the shoulders. *To stay in neutral, imagine there is an egg lying under your* *waist in the gentle curve of your back. As you twist over, be careful not to flatten your lower back and crush it.* Shoulder blades stay down into your back throughout.

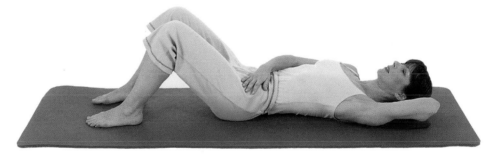

3 **Inhale** and roll back down to Step 1 position keeping the stomach muscles engaged. Repeat Steps 2–3 for required repetitions.

Transition: Take both arms up to the ceiling for the Chest Opener (see page 50).

✓ Lift both shoulders forward, but keep both shoulder blades down into the back as you move.

✓ Ensure the knees don't roll any wider apart.

✓ Relax your head in your hand so there is no tension in the neck.

chest opener

body benefits

- opens the chest and counteracts rounded shoulders

- releases neck and shoulder tension and stiffness in the upper and mid-back

- strengthens and tones the chest and arms

repetitions: 6–10

modifications

If your shoulders are very tight, decrease the range of movement to begin with and just open the arms halfway.

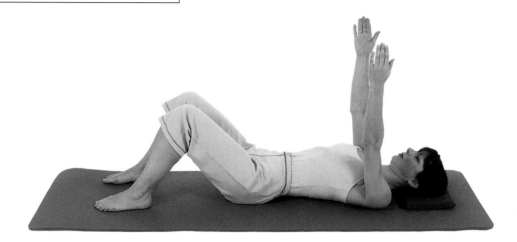

1 Lie on your back with your knees bent at a 90-degree angle, feet hip-width apart. Make sure you are in neutral spine with your neck and shoulders relaxed. Lift both arms to the ceiling, shoulder-width apart, with your palms facing each other. Keep the arms straight without locking your elbows. Your hands should be level with your sternum.

precision points

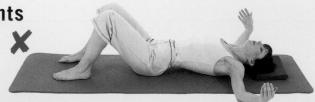

✗ Don't bend your arms.

✗ Don't let your ribs stick out or arch your back as you open your arms.

1 2 3

caution

● Proceed with caution if you are prone to shoulder dislocation.

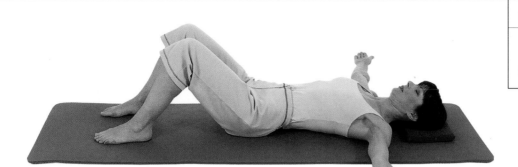

2 **Inhale** as you slowly open your arms straight out to the sides without bending them. Slide your shoulder blades down into your back as the arms open. *Imagine you are painting the arc of a rainbow beginning at the center and working your way outward to each end.*

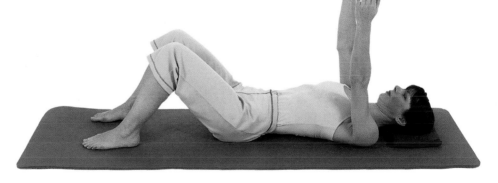

3 **Exhale**, drawing in the abdominals, to return your arms to the starting position, using your chest muscles to perform the movement.

Transition: Turn your palms away from you to prepare for the Arm Splits (see page 52).

✓Open your arms to a T-position. Don't allow your arms to move up to the top of your shoulders or to chin level as this can create tension.

✓Keep your shoulder blades down into your back as you open your arms.

arm splits

body benefits

- strengthens and tones the back, chest, and arm muscles

- releases tension in the neck, shoulders, and upper back

- stretches the chest muscles to counteract round shoulders.

repetitions: 6–10 each way

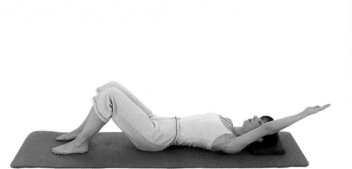

2 **Exhale**, drawing in the abdominals, and split one arm in each direction so that your upper arm moves toward ear level, while you take your lower arm to hip level. Make sure your shoulder blades slide down into your back as you move, keeping the tops of your shoulders away from your ears. *Imagine your arms opening and closing like scissors.*

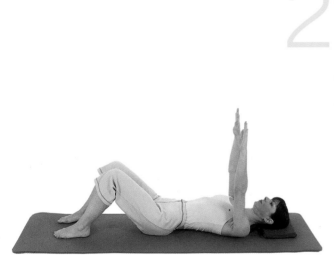

1 Lie on your back with your knees bent at a 90-degree angle, feet hip-width apart. Reach your arms up to the ceiling. Your arms are straight without locking your elbows, with your palms facing away from you. **Inhale**.

precision points

✗ Don't bend your arms or lift your shoulders toward your ears.

✗ Don't arch your back or lift your ribcage as you move.

1 2 3

caution

● If you have a recent shoulder injury, check with your doctor first, and go slowly and carefully on this one.

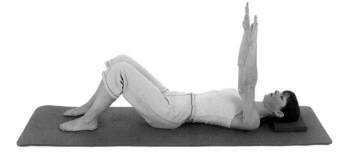

3 **Inhale** to return your arms to the starting position.

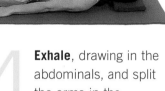

4 **Exhale**, drawing in the abdominals, and split the arms in the opposite direction.

modifications

If your shoulders are very tight, or the movement is uncomfortable, try reducing the range of movement and just take your arms halfway in each direction until you grow more flexible.

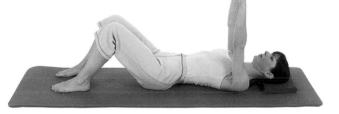

5 **Inhale** to return your arms to the ceiling.

Transition: Take your arms to your sides, straighten your legs out, and roll on to your side for the Double Leg Lift (see page 54). Or take your arms to your sides, roll onto your side, and press yourself up with your hands to come to a sitting position for the Roll Down (see page 76).

✓ Only take your upper arm back as far as you can while ensuring your shoulder blades stay down into your back and that your elbow doesn't bend.

✓ Go for quality of movement rather than trying to force your arm too low so that the tops of your shoulders lift up and your forearm bends.

double leg lift

body benefits

- strengthens the abdominal muscles

- trims the waist

- firms the inner thighs

repetitions: 6–10 each side

modifications

If this position feels uncomfortable for your neck and shoulders, bend your lower arm slightly and place a cushion between your upper arm and head.

If you find it difficult to stop your hips from rolling, lie on your side with your back against a wall to begin with to ensure your hips and shoulders stay square.

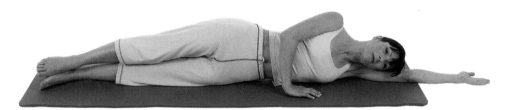

1 Lie on your side with one hip carefully stacked on top of the other. Your ear, the middle of your shoulder, your hip, and your ankle should all be in a straight line. Your feet are pointing down. Your upper arm rests on the floor in front of you, your lower arm stretches out above your head, palm up, your head resting on your arm. Now take your legs slightly further forward. **Inhale**.

precision points

✗

✗ **Don't roll your hips or shoulders forward.**

✗ **Don't collapse at the waist.**

① ② ③

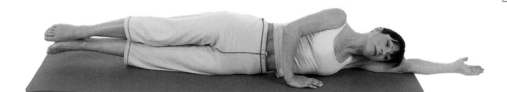

2 **Exhale**, drawing in the abdominals to stabilize your body, and lift both straight legs off the mat—about 4 in (10 cm), squeezing your inner thighs together as you lift, and stretching your legs away from you. *Imagine your inner thighs have been stuck together with glue so they move as a single unit.* Hold for a count of three.

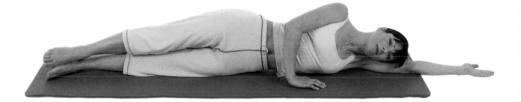

3 **Inhale** as you slowly lower both legs down.

Transition: Bend your lower leg forward for the Outer Thigh Lift (see page 56), or turn your legs out for the Side Kick (see page 118). To save you from switching back and forth from one side to the other while you complete the side-lying leg series that follows, you can perform all the side-lying exercises on one side before rolling over to your other side to repeat them in order on the other side.

✓Keep your torso still. Don't arch your lower back or twist your pelvis or shoulders.

✓Be careful not to shorten your waist. If you stretch your legs away from you, there should be a small gap between your waist and the mat— maintain this throughout.

✓Squeeze your inner thighs together as you lift.

outer thigh lift

body benefits

- tones the outer thigh muscles to reduce saddlebags and create slimmer thighs

- strengthens the buttock muscles

- stretches the leg muscles all the way from your bottom right down to your ankles

repetitions: 6–10 each side

modifications

If you find it uncomfortable lying on your straight arm, bend the arm slightly and place a cushion under your head.

If you find it difficult to get a good alignment, lie with your back against a wall to ensure your hips and shoulders stay square.

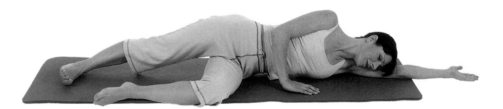

1 Lie on your side with one hip carefully stacked on top of the other. Your ear, the middle of your shoulder, your hip, and your ankle should all be in a straight line. Your feet are pointing down. Your upper arm rests on the floor in front of you, the lower arm stretches out above your head, palm up, your head resting on your arm. Bend your lower leg forward to give a little more support. Reach your upper leg away from you without moving your hips, and flex your foot. Turn the thigh of the upper leg inward in the hip socket so that the leg is slightly internally rotated, without actually moving the hip itself. **Inhale**.

precision points

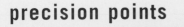

✗ Don't allow the small of your waist to collapse into the floor.

✗ Don't allow your hip to roll forward as you lift your top leg to hip height.

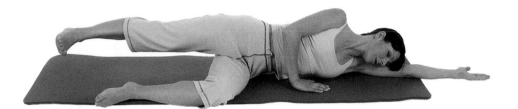

2 **Exhale**, drawing in the abdominals to keep your body stable and squeezing your buttock muscles gently together, stretch the upper leg away from you, as you lift it level with the hip. Lengthen your waist and really reach your upper leg away from you, keeping the internal rotation, pushing through the heel of your foot as you lift. *Imagine you are trying to touch the wall opposite you with your heel.*

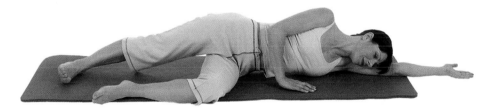

3 **Inhale** and lower your leg to your starting position.

Transition: Straighten your lower leg and cross your upper leg over it for the Inner Thigh Lift (see page 58).

✓ Your lower ribs should remain still and not push forward.

✓ The alignment of your body is vital in this exercise. Keep your body in a straight line with your hips facing forward. Don't let them roll forward or backward as you move.

✓ Keep the foot flexed throughout. If you have internally rotated your thigh in the hip socket correctly, your heel will be slightly higher than your toes.

inner thigh lift

body benefits

- strengthens and firms the inner thigh muscles

repetitions: 6–10 each side

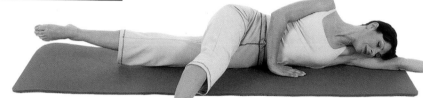

2 **Exhale**, drawing in the abdominals, and stretch your lower leg away from you as you slowly lift the heel about 6 in (15 cm) off the mat. Make sure you keep your lower knee facing forward throughout and that your hips don't move. *Imagine that you are trying to touch the wall opposite you with your heel.*

1 Lie on your side with one hip carefully stacked on top of the other. Your ear, the middle of your shoulder, your hip, and your ankle should all be in a straight line. Your feet are pointing down. Your upper arm rests on the floor in front of you, your lower arm stretches out above your head, palm up, your head resting on your arm. Bring your top leg in front of you so that the foot of your upper leg rests on the floor keeping the leg straight and one hip stacked on top of the other. Your lower leg remains straight underneath it. **Inhale**.

precision points

✘ Don't bend your leg.

✘ Don't allow your hips to roll forward or back.

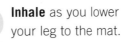

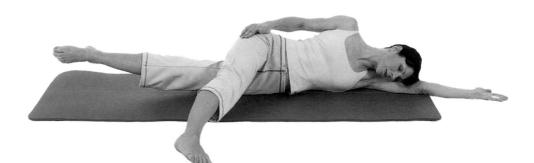

3 **Inhale** as you lower your leg to the mat.

Transition: After completing the inner thigh lift on both sides, roll onto your front for the Hamstring Lift (see page 60), or the Single Leg Kick (see page 120).

modifications

If you find this uncomfortable for your shoulders, bend your lower arm slightly and rest a cushion on top of your arm on which to rest your head.

If it is difficult to keep your back and hips stable, or your top leg straight, perform this exercise with your back against a wall, bend your top leg and rest it on two pillows to stabilize your hips.

To ensure that your hip doesn't move and that you concentrate the work on the inner thigh, place your upper hand just below your hip and gently press down toward the mat.

✓ **Make sure that the hip, knee, and foot of the lower leg face forward.**

✓ **Keep your torso still.**

✓ **Think of pushing through the heel of your lower foot to lengthen the leg away from you as you lift. You should feel the inner thigh working to lift your leg up.**

✓ **Keep the whole movement slow and smooth.**

hamstring lift

body benefits

- lifts and tones the buttocks

- strengthens the hamstring muscles in the back of the thighs

- stretches the legs for a more stream- lined appearance

repetitions: 6–10 on each leg

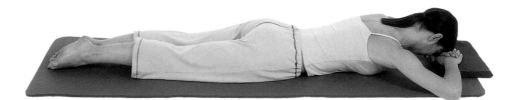

1 Lie on your front with your legs stretched away from you, feet together. Bend your elbows and place your hands one on top of the other under your forehead. Press your pubic bone gently toward the mat to lengthen your lower back. **Inhale**.

precision points

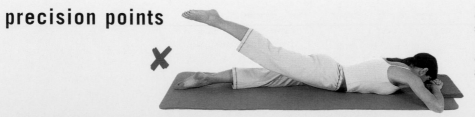

✗ Don't lift your shoulders.

✗ Don't lift your hips along with your leg.

1 2 3

caution

● You should feel no strain in your lower back.

● Proceed only under supervision if you have a lower back injury.

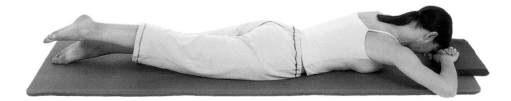

2 **Exhale**, drawing in the abdominals, and lift one leg off the mat, stretching the leg along its length from where it meets the buttock all the way down to the heel. Hold for a count of six. *Imagine your leg is like a piece of sticky toffee, growing thinner and thinner as you stretch it in opposite directions.*

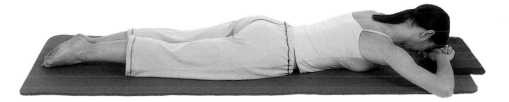

3 **Inhale** and lower your leg.

Transition: Place your arms by your sides and rest your forehead on the head rest for the Arrow (see page 62).

✓To protect your lower back, ensure you keep the abdominals pulled in as you lift so that your lower abdomen pulls away from the floor.

✓Think of pushing your heel away from you to touch the wall opposite, to really lengthen the leg.

✓Lengthen the back of your neck and relax your shoulders throughout.

arrow

---

body benefits

- back and abdominal muscles are strengthened and in time this will help with lower back aches and pains

- helps to improve shoulder stabilization

repetitions: 6–10

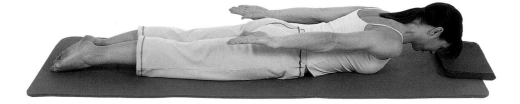

2 **Exhale**, drawing in the abdominals, as you lift your palms toward the ceiling, sliding your shoulder blades down your back toward your hips and lifting your sternum and head and shoulders off the mat. Hold this position for a count of three. *Imagine your body as a streamlined arrow.* Press the crown of your head away from you to keep the back of your neck lengthened and to stretch your spine. At the same time, reach your fingertips in the opposite direction.

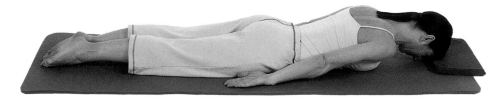

1 Lie facedown on the mat with your arms by your sides, palms up, and fingers pointing toward your feet. Press your pubic bone gently into the mat to keep your lower back long. **Inhale**.

---

precision points

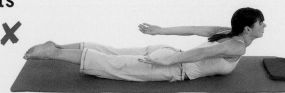

✗ Don't lift your legs.

✗ Don't crunch the back of the neck or look forward instead of down at the mat.

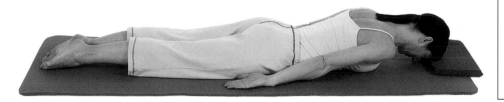

① ② ③

caution

● Proceed with extreme caution and only under supervision if you have any kind of back injury or back condition such as spondylolisthesis.

3 **Inhale** and lower your body down.

Transition: Press your palms down on the mat in front of you and push yourself back so that

your bottom rests on your heels for the Rest Position (see below).

rest position

body benefits

● a great opportunity to cool down toward the end of your session and to stretch your lower back

caution

● If you have problems with your knees, omit the Rest Position and curl into a ball, lying on your side instead.

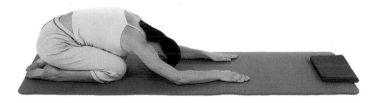

1 From the Arrow position draw your body back so that you are sitting back on

your heels with your arms stretched out in front of you. Rest here for about 30 seconds.

Transition: Slowly roll back up to a kneeling position, coming up one vertebra at a time.

Sit on the mat and then roll down onto your back for the Hamstring Stretch (see page 64).

✓Think of this more as a long stretch than a lift. Don't bring your arms or your body too high off the floor. When your arms lift, the palms should come just above the top of your

buttocks. Your head lifts about 4 in (10 cm) off the mat. You are then resting on your ribs, pubic bone, hipbones, and legs.

✓Keep your abdominals lifted throughout to support your spine.

✓Make sure you lengthen through the back of your neck throughout.

hamstring stretch

body benefits

- lengthens the hamstring muscles in the back of the thighs

- helps to release a tight lower back

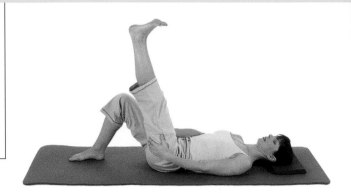

2 **Exhale**, drawing in the abdominals, as you stretch your raised leg up toward the ceiling using your hands to support your leg as it extends. Flex the foot. Hold this for about 30 seconds. Repeat on the other leg.

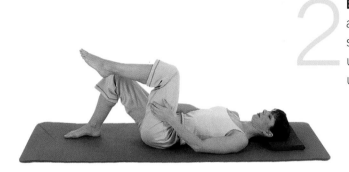

1 Lie on your back with your knees bent and feet hip-width apart. Raise one leg and place your hands behind your thigh to support it. **Inhale**, making sure your tailbone is down on the mat.

modifications

If this position is uncomfortable for you, use a belt or dressing-gown cord to support your foot.

If you have fairly flexible hamstrings, you can stretch the leg that isn't supported by your hands away from you along the mat so that the leg lies straight rather than bent.

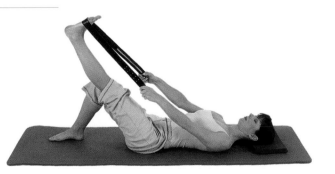

precision points

✗ Don't get carried away with this stretch. Ensure you keep your tailbone down throughout so that the pelvis doesn't tilt even if this means not taking the leg as high.

✓ Think of stretching your raised leg in two directions: the heel up toward the ceiling, but also the other end of the leg, near the buttocks, down into the floor.

✓ Remember to keep your shoulders relaxed and your head on the head rest.

quadriceps stretch

① ② ③

body benefits

● lengthens the quadriceps muscles in the front of the thighs

caution

● Proceed with caution if you have problem knees and omit this exercise if it feels uncomfortable.

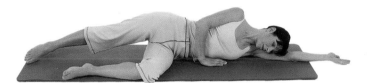

1 Lie on your side in a straight line, with your lower arm above your head, palm up, with the head resting on your arm. Bend your lower leg forward to support you. The higher up you can place this bent leg, the better the muscles will stretch. **Inhale**.

2 **Exhale**, drawing in the abdominals, and reach down to take hold of the ankle of your upper leg and draw it behind you toward your buttocks. You will feel your quadriceps muscle in the front of your thigh stretching. Hold the stretch for 30 seconds, keeping your abdominal muscles engaged. Roll over onto your other side and repeat.

precision points

✗ Don't arch your back and don't roll your body forward or backward.

✓ Gently push your hips forward a little to increase the stretch.

buttock stretch

body benefits

● stretches the buttock muscles

● helps to release a tight lower back

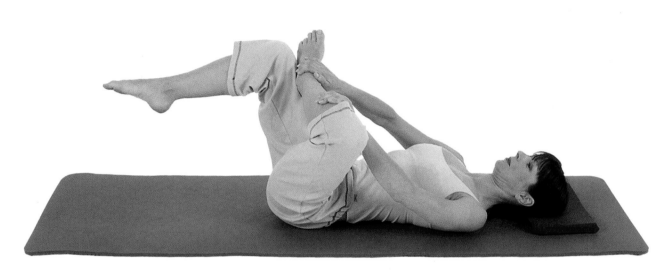

1 Lie down on your back with one knee bent at a 90-degree angle. Cross your other leg over and place the ankle just above the knee. Hold this ankle while keeping your head on the floor. **Inhale**.

precision points

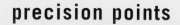

✗ **Don't twist your hips.**

✗ **Don't lift your shoulders or your tailbone.**

caution

● If you have problem knees and this position causes discomfort, omit this exercise for the moment.

2 **Exhale**, drawing in the abdominals, as you pull your top ankle up toward you a little. You will feel a stretch in the buttock of the leg being held at the ankle. Hold this position for about 30 seconds. Repeat with your other leg.

modifications

If this feels relatively easy and you would like to increase the stretch, hold both hands behind the thigh of the leg bent at right angles and bring your knee in a little further toward the chest, still keeping the tailbone down. Hold for 30 seconds on each side.

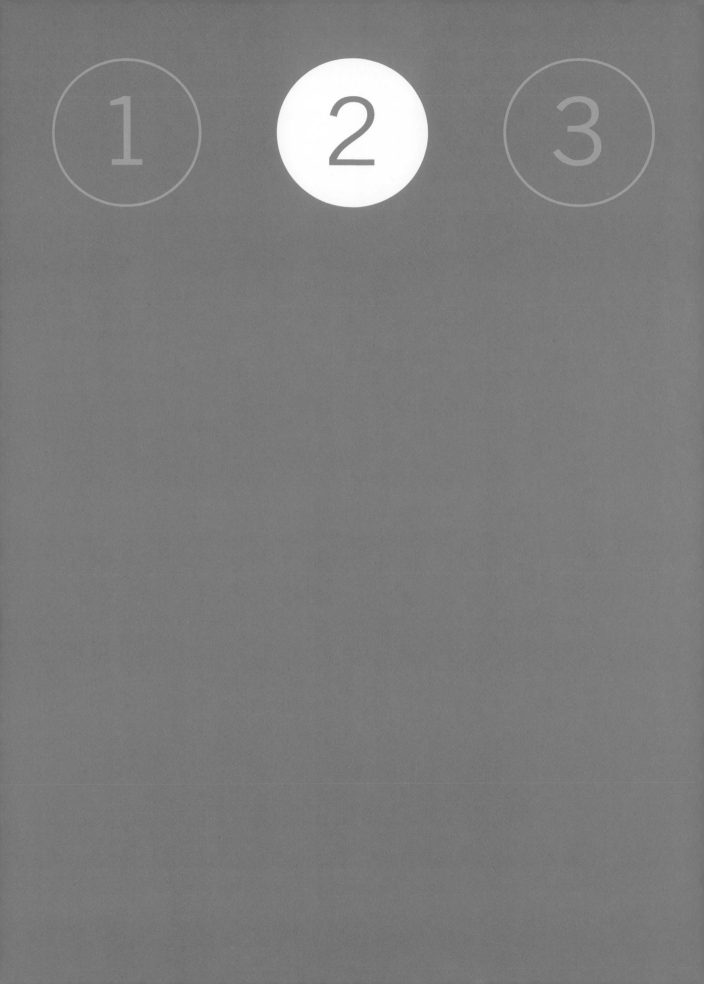

see the difference

benefits after 20 sessions

Practice Pilates for approximately twenty sessions and you will actually *see* the difference:
- Your muscles will be firmer and will have a more toned appearance.
- Your abdominal muscles will strengthen and your stomach will begin to look flatter.
- Your thighs will firm up and should start to look a little slimmer.

As you learn to stretch your muscles, your general flexibility will improve. After twenty sessions, you should see yourself reaching further in your stretches:
- Your spine and hamstrings will be more supple.
- You will be able to peel your spine off the mat more fluidly.
- If you try to touch your toes, the tips of your fingers will probably reach nearer the floor than they used to.

- After twenty sessions, you will look a lot more comfortable in your body. Years of stored tension is releasing and you will move with newfound grace. Your hip joints, knee joints, shoulder joints, and ankle joints will all be freer, and your balance and coordination will improve. Your skin will look clearer, and you will feel less stressed, more focused, and ready to face the world.

- Build regular Pilates practice into your life and the results will speak for themselves. You may find you start receiving compliments on how much younger, fitter, and more relaxed you look. You will no doubt feel better about your body than you have in years. You will have a lot more energy and your confidence will positively soar. You will look and feel more attractive. And, of course, the happier you are, the more people are drawn to you.

level 2 program

You can now perform Level 1 exercises comfortably and correctly and feel ready to move on to Level 2. Practice the Level 2 sequence of exercises three times per week, preferably exercising with one day's rest in between each session. Work your way through them in the order given according to the **Exercise Sequence Chart** (see pages 72–73), adding two to three new ones each time you practice, and skipping over the other new ones for the moment.

Most of the exercises you learned in Level 1 are repeated in your workout for Level 2. There are also some additional exercises, which will feel more complex as you are going to be working several parts of the body simultaneously. The key is to perform the movements slowly and carefully. Review the six fundamental **Pilates principles** (see pages 12–13) and each time you do a workout, pick one of the principles to focus on as you go through the exercises to improve your technique.

The exercises should be performed in the order given here to best balance your body, so start at the beginning and work your way through, leaving out any that you don't yet feel ready for, or if any injury or medical condition prevents you from performing them.

progress at your own pace

Knowing when you are ready to add a new exercise is a choice you must make based on your individual physical strengths and weaknesses. Make sure you are always working within your range. As you attempt a new exercise, listen to your body. For example, if your hamstrings and lower back are tight, the Single Leg Circles (see page 78) may be difficult for you at first. Try the modified version instead until they lengthen out. You need to judge for yourself if any exercises are uncomfortable for you and if you are pushing yourself beyond your limits. If in any doubt, book

a private session with a Pilates teacher and get them to run through the program with you. The key is to listen to your body when trying a new movement. You should feel you are working hard but you should never feel any strain. Just go slowly, enjoy the movement, and use precision and control. Use the transitions too, to ensure that you flow smoothly from one exercise to the next.

Most important, don't rush it. Give yourself plenty of time at this level to ensure you are comfortable with the exercises and performing them correctly before going on to Level 3. Assess yourself continuously to see how you are doing: as long as you're feeling comfortably challenged, you're getting the benefits. There is no point moving up a level quicker than you should. Firstly, it's dangerous and could cause you to strain or injure yourself. Secondly, if you're not performing the exercise correctly because you aren't yet strong enough or flexible enough to do so, you won't get the body improvement. Pay attention to your body and make sure you're giving it the exact level of exercise it needs.

Practice Pilates approximately twenty times at the level that's right for your body and you'll really begin to see a difference.

level 2: exercise sequence char

This exercise chart contains most of the exercises that you learned in Level 1 plus many new ones. Add two to three new ones each time you practice until you have learned the whole sequence. As before, each exercise ends with transition instructions so you can flow smoothly from one exercise to the next.

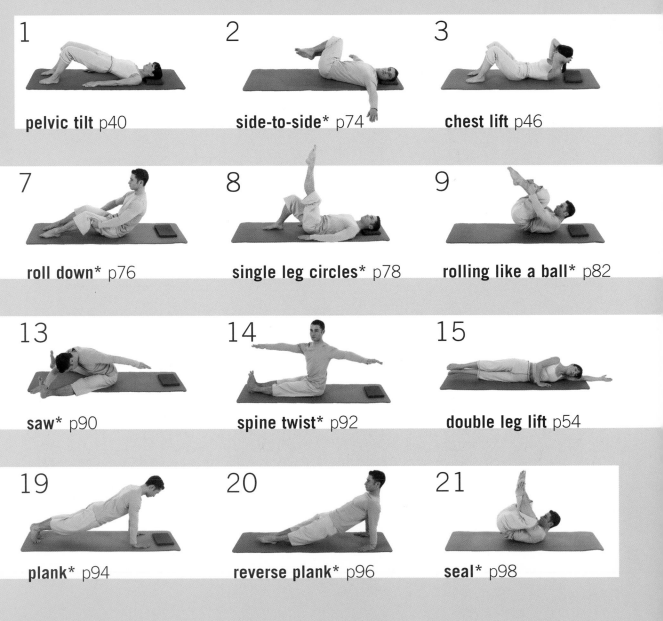

1
pelvic tilt p40

2
side-to-side* p74

3
chest lift p46

7
roll down* p76

8
single leg circles* p78

9
rolling like a ball* p82

13
saw* p90

14
spine twist* p92

15
double leg lift p54

19
plank* p94

20
reverse plank* p96

21
seal* p98

* new exercises

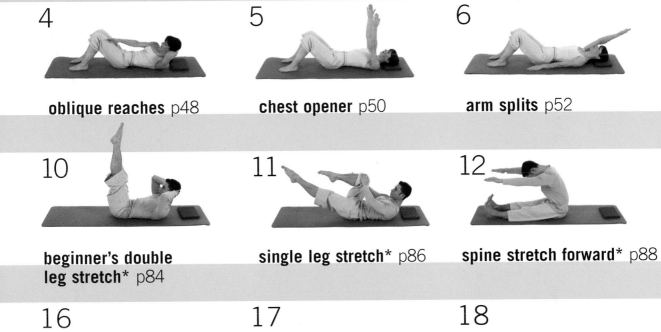

4

oblique reaches p48

5

chest opener p50

6

arm splits p52

10

beginner's double leg stretch* p84

11

single leg stretch* p86

12

spine stretch forward* p88

16

outer thigh lift p56

17

inner thigh lift p58

18

arrow (+ rest position) p62

side-to-side

body benefits

- strengthens the abdominal muscles

- trims the waist

- increases spinal flexibility

repetitions: 5 each side, alternating sides

3 **Exhale**, drawing in the abdominals to bring your knees and head back to center. Relax your thighs. *Imagine your legs are heavy and that you are using purely abdominal strength to bring the knees back.*

2 **Inhale**, keeping the abdominals engaged to support your spine and take your knees over to one side, keeping your shoulder blades firmly on the mat. Turn your head gently to the opposite side.

1 Lie on your back with your knees bent and stretch your arms out to the sides at shoulder height with the palms facing down. Bend your knees in toward your chest. Your knees point to the ceiling and your knees and inner thighs are squeezed tightly together. **Inhale**, then **exhale**, drawing in the abdominal muscles.

precision points

✗ Don't twist your hips or bring your knees further over than your feet.

✗ Don't crunch your neck and lift your shoulders.

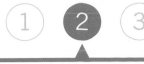

caution

● Proceed only under supervision if you have a back or neck injury.

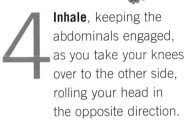

4 **Inhale**, keeping the abdominals engaged, as you take your knees over to the other side, rolling your head in the opposite direction.

5 **Exhale**, drawing in the abdominals to return to center.

Transition: Place the feet back on to the mat, with the knees bent at a 90-degree angle, and feet hip-width apart. Take the arms behind the head for the Chest Lift (see page 46).

modifications

If you feel any tension in your lower back, or if this exercises feels too much for your abdominal muscles, replace it with both the Small Hip Roll (see page 42) and the Hip Roll (see page 44) exercises in Level 1 until your body grows stronger.

✓Relax your neck, chest, and shoulders

✓Keep your shoulder blades down on the mat throughout.

✓Press your palms into the mat for extra stability.

✓Make sure you take your knees and feet directly over to the side without twisting your hips.

✓Your knees and feet should move over to the side as a single unit.

roll down

body benefits

- strengthens the abdominal muscles

- stretches the back to improve flexibility

- encourages good spinal articulation

repetitions: 3–5

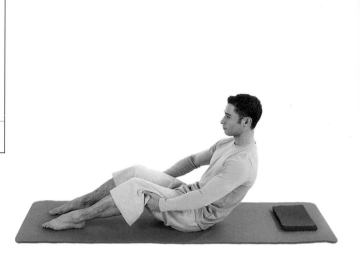

2 **Exhale**, drawing in the abdominals, and curl your tailbone under you, aiming your lower back for the mat so that your spine forms a C-shaped curve. As you **continue to exhale**, keep drawing in the abdominals and try to increase the C-curve by rolling your spine down one vertebra at a time. Roll as far down as your arms will allow without your hands coming away from your thighs. Your shoulder blades stay down into your back. **Inhale** and rest in the C-curve position.

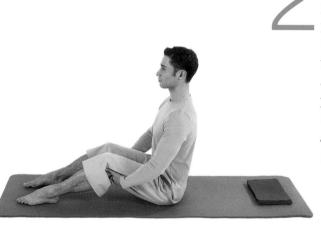

1 Sit up tall with a straight back, with your knees bent at a 90-degree angle and feet hip-width apart. Place your feet as flat as possible. Place your hands around the back of your thighs and lift your elbows wide. **Inhale**.

precision points

✗ Don't allow your ribs to lift or your abdominals to bulge.

✗ Don't straighten your back as you move; it should be curved.

① ② ③

caution

● Omit this exercise if you feel any tension in your lower back.

● Hold your legs lightly if you have weak wrists, elbows, or shoulders.

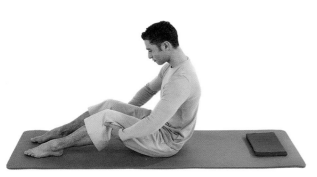

3 **Exhale**, drawing in the abdominals deeper and deeper, to curl back up one vertebra at a time, keeping the C-curve all the way up until your shoulders are above your hips. *Imagine your abdominals are being drawn back toward your spine by a supermagnetic force.*

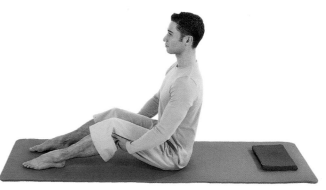

4 **Inhale** and sit up tall again with a straight back.

Transition: Lower yourself down to the mat with your arms by your sides for the Single Leg Circles (see page 78).

modifications

Keep your feet flat on the mat, if possible. If this is uncomfortable, lift the toes but keep your heels on the mat.

✓ **Be careful not to lean your body back. Instead, use your abdominals so the movement begins from the base of your spine.**

✓ **Keep the abdominal muscles drawing in to curve your lower back.**

✓ **Keep your shoulder blades down into your back and your elbows lifted.**

single leg circles

body benefits

- increases strength and flexibility in the hips

- lengthens the back of the thighs

- strengthens the inner thighs

- stretches and strengthens the outer thighs

- firms the buttocks

repetitions: 5 circles in each direction with one leg, 5 circles in each direction with the other leg.

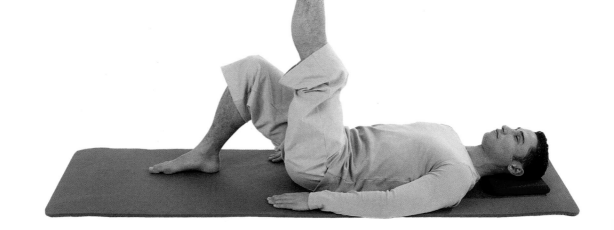

1 Lie on your back with your knees bent at a 90-degree angle, feet hip-width apart. Place your arms by your sides, pressing your palms down into the mat for support. Ensure that the back of your neck is lengthened and your shoulders are down and relaxed. Lift one leg straight up to the ceiling, turning out the leg (see page 27) by engaging the lower buttock muscles to rotate the thigh outward in the hip socket. Your inner thigh also engages. Point your toe. Your other leg remains bent with the foot firmly planted on the mat.

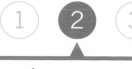

① ② ③

caution

● Proceed only under supervision if you have a back injury.

● If you experience any clicking in your hip, try bending your knee slightly and reducing the size of the circle.

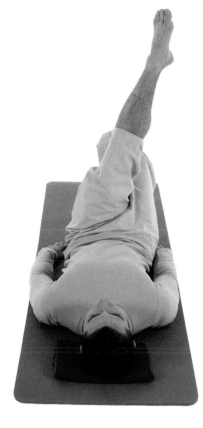

2 **Inhale** as you cross your leg over your body without letting your hips lift off the mat.

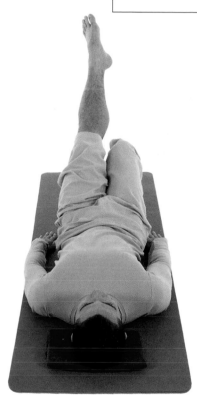

3 **Exhale**, drawing in the abdominals, as you sweep your leg in a circle down toward the mid-line of your body.

single leg circles cont.

4 Keep **exhaling** as you continue the circle round to the other side of your body.

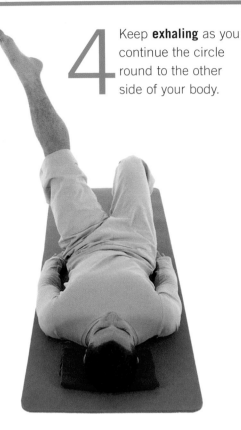

5 Then circle your leg back up to its starting position in the center, still **exhaling**. *Imagine you are painting a small circle in the air, using your big toe as the paintbrush.* Control the movement with your abdominals so that your torso and your bent leg stay completely still throughout. Repeat 5 times.

precision points

✗

✗ Don't lift the pelvis.

✗ Don't crunch the neck and shoulders.

6

Reverse the circle by **inhaling** to take your leg over to the side away from your body. **Exhale** as you take the leg down, around, and back to the center. Repeat 5 times.

Transition: Place both feet back on the mat, knees bent, then roll onto one side and push yourself up with your hands to come up to sitting for Rolling Like a Ball (see page 82).

Or, if you are able, lower your raised leg, take your arms above your head, and perform a Roll Up (see page 108) to bring you up to sitting position for Rolling Like a Ball.

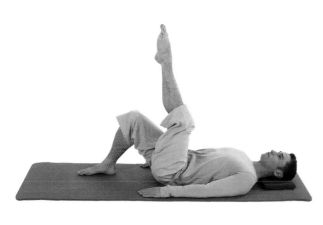
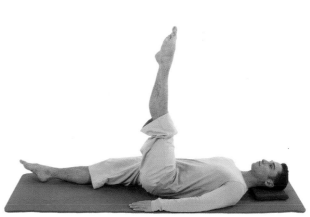

modifications

If you have a tight lower back and hamstrings, holding the position may feel a little difficult. If you are unable to keep both hips down on the mat while straightening the leg to the ceiling, bend the knee slightly until you are able to straighten the leg out comfortably.

Once you can perform the Single Leg Circles while keeping your torso stable when the lower knee is bent, you can challenge yourself further by straightening this leg along the mat.

Once you can perform the movement while keeping your torso completely stable, challenge yourself further by increasing the size of the circle without sacrificing your core stability.

✓ **Ensure that your body remains still while you circle your leg in your hip joint so that you don't roll off to one side and your back does not arch.**

✓ **In order to stop your quadriceps from doing all the work, keep your thigh turned out slightly in the hip and think of using your buttock to help make the movement.**

✓ **Your toes reach for the ceiling as you circle to keep your leg completely straight.**

✓ **The emphasis of this movement is on the "upswing."**

rolling like a ball

body benefits

- strengthens the abdominals

- massages the spine and improves spinal flexibility

- improves balance and control

repetitions: 6–10

2 **Inhale** as you roll back on the mat to the base of your shoulder blades, keeping your rounded shape. Feel your spine roll back onto the mat one vertebra at a time so that you end up with your bottom toward the ceiling. *Imagine you are running up the scale on a piano as you try to feel each vertebra connecting with the mat.*

1 Sit near the front of your mat with your feet together and knees bent. Take hold of one ankle in each hand with elbows wide to the sides. Pull your feet close to your buttocks and roll your head down toward your knees. Open your knees slightly. Rock back fractionally so that your back is rounded and you are balancing on your tailbone with your feet just lifted off the floor. You want to keep this rounded ball shape throughout.

precision points

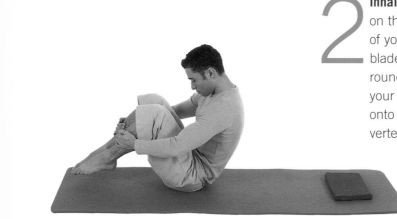

✗ Don't move your feet away from your buttocks. Keep a tight ball shape.

✗ Don't let your head touch the mat.

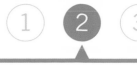

3 **Exhale**, drawing in the abdominals, to roll back up to your starting position so that you are balancing on your tailbone again, keeping a rounded spine. Your feet hover just above the ground. Keep your shoulder blades down into your back throughout.

Transition: From sitting, roll down to the mat one vertebra at a time, and draw the knees toward the chest to prepare for the Beginner's Double Leg Stretch (see page 84).

modifications

Don't worry if you can't roll all the way back up initially, just roll up as high as you can and continue to practice.

If the exercise feels very difficult, place one hand behind each thigh instead, elbows wide. Still keep the feet together, the knees slightly open, and the lower back curved. Try rolling in this position.

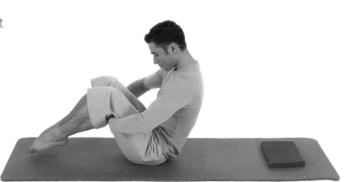

✓ **Keep your shoulders relaxed and down throughout. Don't let them creep up around your ears.**

✓ **Keep your head toward your knees, especially when rolling up.**

✓ **Once you've found the movement, try not to use too much momentum. Instead use your abdominal strength to get you back up.**

✓ **Keep your lower back curved throughout, so that you don't straighten your back at the balance point, in particular.**

beginner's double leg stretch

body benefits

- strengthens the abdominals

- strengthens the leg muscles

repetitions: 6–10

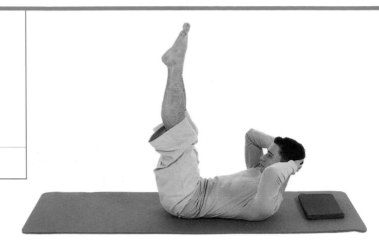

2 Continue this exhalation as you straighten your legs toward the ceiling, pointing your toes. *Imagine your back is glued to the floor.*

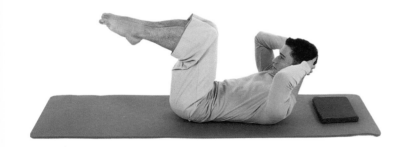

1 Lie on your back with your knees bent and shins parallel to the floor; your knees are at a 90-degree angle to your torso. Interlace your fingers and place your hands behind your head with your head resting on the mat. Your elbows are wide but should just be within your peripheral vision. **Inhale**, then **exhale** slowly, drawing in your abdominals, and rolling your head and shoulders off the mat, hinging at the breastbone as you slide your shoulder blades down your back.

precision points

✗

✗ **Don't allow your elbows to fall inward.**

✗ **Don't arch your back.**

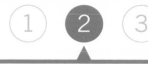

caution

● Proceed only under supervision if you have a neck or back injury.

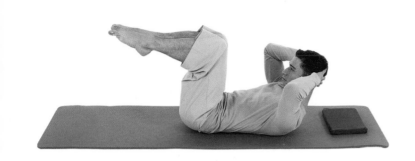

3 **Inhale** and rebend your knees with your abdominal muscles still engaged.

4 **Exhale**, drawing in the abdominals, as you roll your head back onto the mat.

Transition: Rest both hands lightly on one knee for the Single Leg Stretch (see page 86).

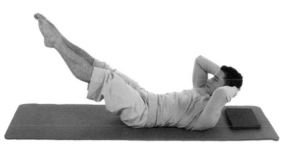

modifications

If you can't fully straighten your legs to the ceiling, straighten them as far as you can, and perform the exercise with the legs slightly bent.

Once you are comfortable performing the exercise with the legs straight, you can begin to lower your straight legs to an angle of 45 degrees. If your back starts to arch off the mat, you have taken the legs too low.

✓ Let your head be heavy in your hands. Use your abdominals to lift so there is no strain in the neck.

✓ Keep the elbows wide and the shoulders relaxed.

✓ Keep your back flat on the mat throughout.

single leg stretch

body benefits

- tones the abdominal muscles

- trims the waist

- encourages good body alignment

repetitions: 6–10 each side, alternating legs

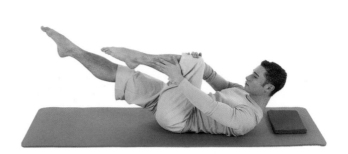

3 **Exhale**, drawing in the abdominals as you straighten one leg at a 45-degree angle. Your torso and your other leg, supported by your two hands, don't move. You are now in the starting position. *Imagine your torso is frozen in ice and cannot move.* **Inhale**.

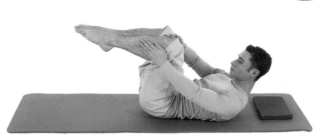

2 **Inhale**, keeping the abdominals engaged, and roll your head and shoulders off the mat, sliding your shoulder blades down into your back.

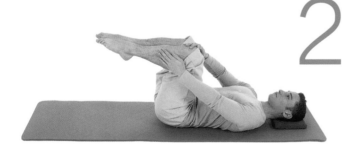

1 Lie on your back with your knees bent and shins parallel to the mat. Place one hand on the inside of your opposite knee. The other hand reaches down the outside of your leg, toward your ankle. Knees are close together. The elbows are wide. **Inhale**, then **exhale**, drawing in the abdominals.

precision points

✗ Don't twist your shoulders and hips.

✗ Don't drop your bent leg.

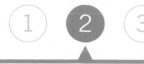

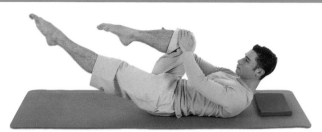

caution

● Proceed only under supervision if you have a back injury.

● Proceed with caution if you have weak knees.

4 Without changing the position of your torso, **exhale** and draw in the abdominals as you switch legs, bending your straight leg in, switching your hands over to that leg, while straightening your other leg out to 45 degrees. Continue to switch legs on each exhalation for the required number of repetitions. Between exhalations, there is the tiniest of in-breaths, almost a "sniff." The focus is on the out-breath as you bend one leg in and straighten the other.

Transition: Take the hands behind the head for the Beginner's Criss-Cross (see page 114). Or roll over onto one side and press yourself up to sitting with your hands to prepare for the Spine Stretch Forward (see page 88).

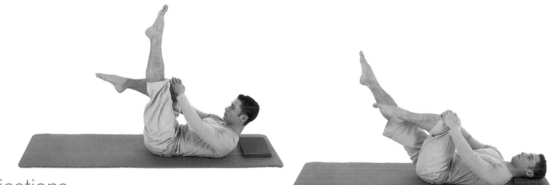

modifications

If you find it difficult to keep your back flat on the mat, try straightening your leg toward the ceiling instead. As your strength improves, bring your leg to a lower angle.

If you feel tension in the neck, perform the leg movements with both hands behind your head, supporting the weight of your head with your hands.

If this still feels tough, rest your head and shoulders on the head rest throughout, placing both hands on one knee.

If your knee aches, hold under the knee instead and take the exercise at a slower pace so there is no pain, or omit it entirely.

✓**Keep your back flat on the mat throughout and your shoulder blades down.**

✓**Pay attention to your hand positions as this keeps you aligned correctly.**

✓**Keep your torso and bent leg completely still as you lengthen the other leg away.**

✓**Watch that your bent leg stays at a 90-degree angle and that your foot and calf don't start to flop toward the floor.**

spine stretch forward

body benefits

- works the abdominal muscles

- a great stretch for the lower back

- improves spinal flexibility

- stretches the back of the legs

- improves sitting posture

repetitions: 3–5

2 **Exhale**, drawing in the abdominals, and round your spine forward one vertebra at a time. Keep rolling forward until your spine forms a letter C-shaped curve. *Imagine your straight back is against a wall. Lower your head, then peel your* *upper back off the wall, followed by your mid-back and finally your lower back.* Try to resist the stretch by drawing in your abdominals as you round forward, stretching your lower back further behind you. Your head should end up just above your arms, following the line of the C-shaped curve.

1 Sit up tall with your legs straight, hip-width apart, and your feet flexed so that your toes point to the ceiling. Lift your arms parallel to your legs at shoulder height, ensuring the shoulder blades are relaxed down into your back. **Inhale**.

precision points

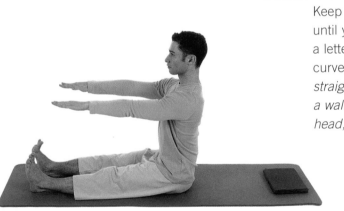

✗ Don't hold your arms too high; they should stay at shoulder height.

✗ Don't hold your back straight as you roll forward.

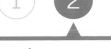

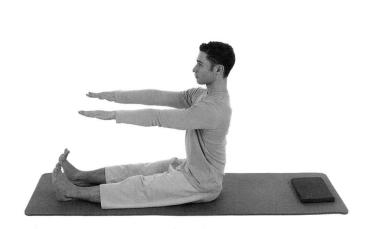

caution

● Proceed only under supervision if you have any kind of back injury.

● Proceed with caution if you have any stiffness in the lower back.

3 **Inhale**, then **exhale**, drawing in your abdominals as you reverse the movement. Roll back up your imaginary wall to your tall sitting position, one vertebra at a time, placing your lower back, then your mid- and then upper back, and finally your head. Keep pulling your abdominals in until you're sitting up really tall. Focus on lifting up out of your hips with a straight back.

Transition: Take your feet just wider than hip-width apart, and reach your arms out to the sides at shoulder height for the Saw (see page 90).

modifications

If the stretch behind your knees is too much, bend your knees slightly so the thigh muscles relax.

If the stretch is too much in your lower back, or you find it hard to sit up tall due to a tight lower back or hamstrings, bend your knees slightly and don't roll down as far. Gradually increase the range of movement as you grow more flexible.

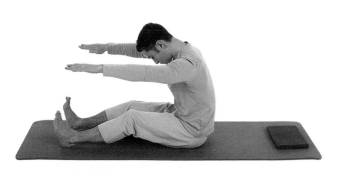

✓ **Keep the space between your ribcage and hips. Imagine you are stretching up and over a beach ball positioned between your legs so you don't collapse your torso as you roll.**

✓ **As you roll, keep your feet flexed and think of pushing through your heels to really feel the stretch in the backs of your legs.**

✓ **Watch that there is no tension in your neck throughout the stretch. Just let your head hang.**

✓ **Roll back up to sit tall, without leaning forward or back, your shoulder blades down into your back, and reaching the crown of your head up to the ceiling.**

saw

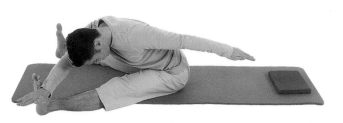

body benefits

- stretches the waist, hips, and back of thighs

- improves spinal rotation

- helps to empty and cleanse the lungs

repetitions: 3–5 each side, alternating sides

3 **Exhale**, drawing in the abdominals, as you round forward, reaching your front arm forward and down, aiming for your little toe. *Imagine you are sawing off your little toe with your little finger.* The back hand sweeps back and lowers to line up with the front hand.

2 **Inhale** and slowly twist your upper body from the waist. Let the arms float with you until your forward arm is directly over your opposite leg. Lengthen your spine up as you twist, keeping your hips and legs glued to the mat.

1 Sit up tall, reaching up through the crown of your head to lengthen your spine up toward the ceiling. Reach your arms out straight to the sides, so that you can just see them within your peripheral vision, with the palms facing down. Your legs are straight, just wider than hip-width apart, with your feet flexed.

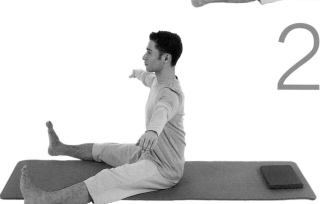

precision points

✗

✗ **Don't allow your hips to roll.**

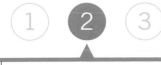

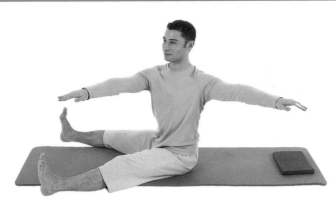

caution

● Omit this exercise if you have a back or neck injury.

4 **Inhale**, remaining on the diagonal as you roll, one vertebra at a time, back to sitting. Initiate this movement from your center. As you come up, lift your arms until they are shoulder height and parallel to the floor.

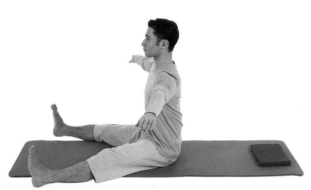

5 **Exhale**, drawing in the abdominals, and twist from the waist back to center and your Step 1 starting position. Repeat, twisting to the other side.

Transition: Bring your straight legs together for the Spine Twist (see page 92).

modifications

If the stretch is too much for the back of your knees, or if you find it hard to sit up straight, bend your knees slightly to give yourself extra lift.

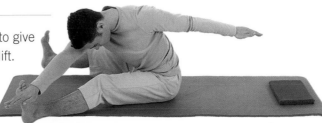

✓ Ensure that you twist from your waist, not from your shoulders or hips. Keep your hipbones facing forward as you twist.

✓ Your head rolls forward with your body and your neck is relaxed.

✓ Roll up through the spine to come back to sitting, don't straighten up with a flat back. Your head should be the last part to come up.

spine twist

body benefits

- stretches the spine

- lengthens the muscles in the back of the legs

- trims the waistline

- wrings stale air from your lungs

repetitions: 5 each side, alternating sides

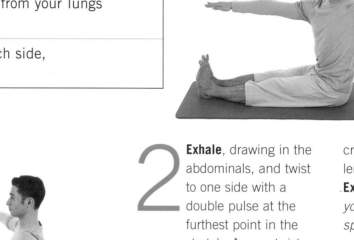

2 **Exhale**, drawing in the abdominals, and twist to one side with a double pulse at the furthest point in the stretch. As you twist, keep your hips still and reach up through the crown of your head to lengthen your spine. **Exhale fully**. *Imagine your are wringing your spine as you twist, as you would wring water from a towel.*

1 Sit up tall with your arms stretched out to the sides. Your palms facedown and your shoulder blades are down into your back throughout. Your arms should lie just within your peripheral vision. Your legs are straight with your thighs squeezed tightly together and your feet flexed so your toes point to the ceiling. **Inhale**.

precision points

✗ Don't twist from your shoulders or let your body fall forward.

✗ Don't allow your heel bones to come out of alignment.

① ② ③

caution

● Omit this exercise if you have back problems.

● If you have a delicate shoulder, only twist as far as you can without any pain.

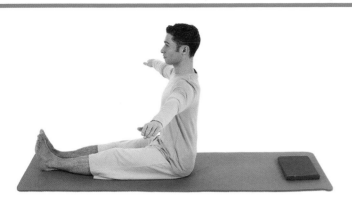

3 **Inhale** to twist back to center.

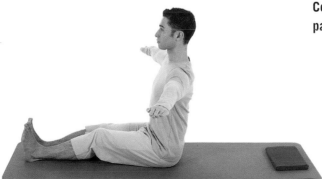

4 **Exhale**, drawing in the abdominals, as you twist to the other side with a double pulse. **Inhale** as you return to center.

Transition: Roll onto one side in a straight line for the Double Leg Lift (see page 54). Or bend your knees and roll down one vertebra at a time so that you are lying on your back to prepare for the Corkscrew (see page 116).

modifications

If you feel too much stress on the backs of your legs, or if you find you can't sit up with a straight spine, bend your knees slightly for more lift.

✓ If you find one heel moves further forward than the other, you are incorrectly moving your hip.

✓ Only twist from your waist, your hipbones remain facing forward throughout.

✓ Allow your head to follow the twist in your spine. Don't overturn the head.

plank

body benefits

- builds upper body strength in particular, but tones and strengthens the whole body

- strengthens back, chest, shoulders, back of thighs, buttocks, abdominal muscles, and arms

repetitions: 3

2 Reach one leg back and place the ball of your foot on the floor, straightening your leg out and putting your weight on it.

1 Kneel on all fours with your hands directly underneath your shoulders. Keep your arms straight, but don't lock your elbows. Knees should be hip-width apart.

precision points

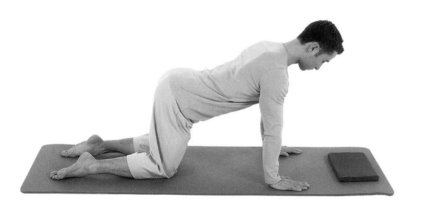

✗ Don't let your hips sink so the diagonal line is lost.

✗ Don't let your shoulders collapse.

1 2 3

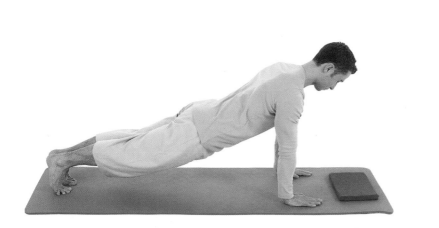

caution

● Omit this exercise if you have a shoulder or elbow injury.

● Omit this exercise if you have weak hands or wrists.

3 Straighten your other leg out to join the first and place your weight evenly between the balls of your two feet. Your feet should be side by side with your legs pressed tightly together. Draw your abdominals up into the body to support the spine throughout. Your arms are straight with your shoulders pressed down away from your ears. Your body forms a plank—a straight line from your shoulders all the way down to your heels. *Imagine you are a rod of steel that cannot sag.* Hold this position for 2–4 breaths. Bend the knees to rest, then repeat twice more.

Transition: Bend the legs in and down to the floor to return to the kneeling position. Turn over and sit up tall with your legs stretched out in front of you to prepare for the Reverse Plank (see page 96).

modifications

If you are not yet strong enough to maintain the plank position, or if you find it is placing strain on your wrists, omit this exercise for the moment.

✓ **Plant your hands and feet firmly into the mat.**

✓ **Lengthen through the crown of your head to keep the back of your neck long. Your neck should be aligned with the rest of your spine. Look down.**

✓ **Squeeze your thighs together and slightly engage your buttocks to maintain your "rod of steel."**

✓ **To keep your pelvis aligned, think of tucking your pubic bone under slightly. Don't allow your bottom to lift or to sink.**

reverse plank

body benefits

- challenges abdominal strength

- firms and strengthens the buttocks and back of thighs

- strengthens the upper torso

repetitions: 3

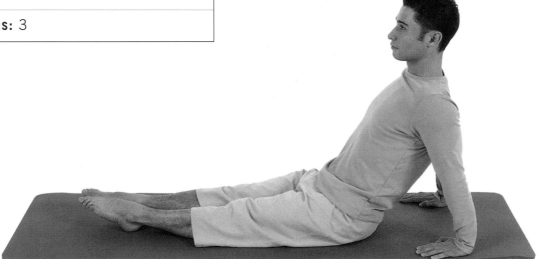

1 Sit up tall with your legs stretched out in front of you and your hands behind you, fingers pointing toward your body. Squeeze your inner thighs together throughout. **Inhale**.

precision points

✘ **Don't allow your hips and shoulders to collapse.**

✘ **Don't throw your head back.**

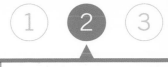

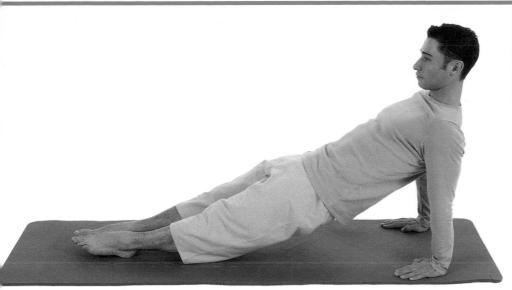

caution

● Omit this exercise if you have a shoulder or elbow injury.

● Omit this exercise if you have weak hands or wrists.

2 **Exhale**, drawing in the abdominals, and press your hips up to the ceiling to establish a reverse plank position. Engage your buttock muscles, and slide your shoulder blades down into your back to hold yourself in one long straight line from shoulders to feet. Look straight ahead. *Imagine you are a rod of steel and cannot sag.* Hold this position for 2–4 breaths. Lower your hips to the mat to rest and repeat twice more.

Transition: Slowly lower your hips and return to Step 1 position. Press your hands into the mat on either side of you and lift yourself forward so that you are sitting at the front of your mat to prepare for the Seal (see page 98).

modifications

If holding this position is uncomfortable on your hands and wrists, try turning your palms out so that your fingers point out to the sides.

If the above modification is still difficult for you, omit this exercise for the moment.

To start with, let your head be positioned so that your eyes look forward. As you progress, try to keep your head and neck aligned with your spine.

✓ **Lengthen the crown of your head up to the ceiling to elongate the back of your neck.**

✓ **Slide your shoulder blades down into your back.**

✓ **Use your abdominals and engage your buttock muscles to keep your hips lifted.**

✓ **Heels remain on the mat even if your toes need to lift slightly.**

seal

body benefits

- fantastic spinal massage

- improves spinal flexibility

- strengthens the abdominal muscles

- improves balance and control

- a great cool-down exercise

repetitions: 5–10

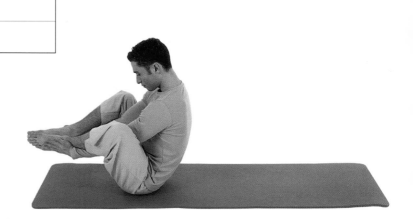

1 Sit at the front of your mat with your knees bent toward your chest and heels together. Open your knees to shoulder width and thread your hands through the legs to hold the outside of your ankles.

Round your back and rock back a fraction so that your feet are just off the mat and you are balancing on your tailbone. Bring your chin slightly toward your chest.

precision points

✘ **Don't lift your shoulders.**

✘ **Don't throw your head back and forth or roll onto your neck.**

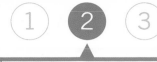

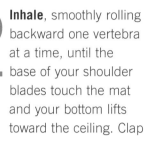

2 **Inhale**, smoothly rolling backward one vertebra at a time, until the base of your shoulder blades touch the mat and your bottom lifts toward the ceiling. Clap your heels together 3 times *like a seal clapping its flippers*, keeping your chin tucked toward your chest.

3 **Exhale**, drawing in your abdominals to roll back up to your balance point at the end of Step 1. Clap your heels together again 3 times.

modifications

If it is difficult to rock back and forth, leave out the claps for now, and just focus on using your abdominals to roll each way. As you get stronger, just add the claps after the forward movement. You can add the claps after the backward movement later.

✓**Focus on balancing at the beginning and end of the movement.**

✓**Use your breath and control of your abdominals to bring you forward and back. Try not to rely on momentum.**

✓**Keep your shoulder blades down your back, and make sure your lower back is curved throughout.**

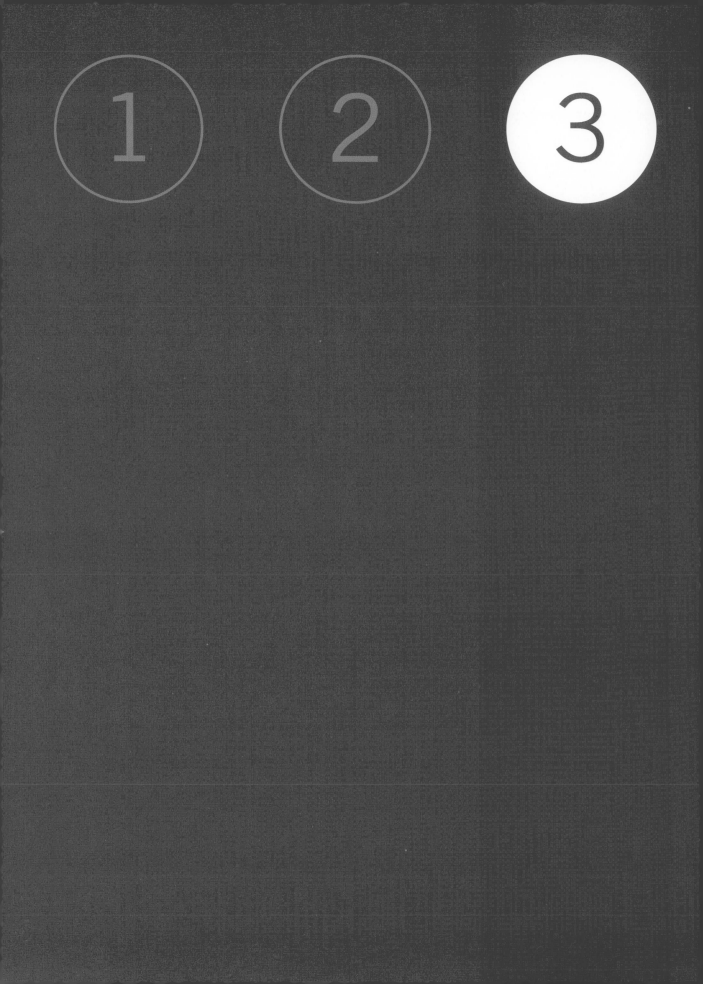

a whole new you

benefits after 30 sessions

Practice Pilates for approximately thirty sessions at the level that is right for your body, and you'll discover a whole new you, a whole new way of moving, and a whole new body shaping up, too.

outer benefits

After thirty sessions performing Pilates correctly, you will see real results:

• You will look stronger and sleeker. You are beginning to rebalance your body, toning up flabby muscles, and stretching out bulky ones.

• Your abdominal muscles will be firmer and flatter, the saddlebags on the outsides of your thighs will slim down, and your inner thighs will be less wobbly.

• Your upper arms will look more toned, your buttocks will be lifted and firmer. You will be the proud owner of a more streamlined shape.

Some people find they go down a clothing size in thirty sessions without actually losing weight. Muscle takes up less space in your body than fat, and after thirty sessions, you will definitely build more muscle. Plus, more lean muscle increases your metabolism (the rate at which you burn off fat). If you also combine this program with a healthy weight-loss plan, you can safely lose up to 20 lbs (10 kg), depending on your body weight.

• With your new flexibility, you will find you can move more freely with fewer aches and pains. Chronically overworked muscles will relax, lower back aches ease, neck and shoulder tension lessen. Your joints will be more mobile and should cause fewer problems.

• You will have much better body awareness and you will improve your alignment. You will discover bad habits and reeducate your body. You will teach yourself a whole new way of moving and develop a much more youthful posture.

inner benefits

• You will feel rested and relaxed, and yet your mind will be more alert and open to new challenges. After all, you face new challenges every time you practice Pilates.

• The overall result will be that your self-esteem will soar to new heights. You will feel much more confident and experience a profound sense of well-being.

• I'm also willing to bet that after 30 sessions, you will have finally found an exercise program you actually enjoy and that you can imagine sustaining for the rest of your life.

level 3 program

By now you have mastered Level 2 exercises and have a good understanding of what the Pilates method is all about. You feel ready and able to take that understanding further and move on to Level 3.

Practice the Level 3 sequence of exercises three times per week, preferably exercising with one day's rest in between each session. Work your way through them in the order given in the **Exercise Sequence Chart** (see pages 104–105), adding one to two new ones each time you practice and skipping the other new ones for the moment.

You are now moving into Intermediate Level Pilates. Many of the exercises you learned in Levels 1 and 2 are repeated in Level 3, but some of them have been modified to make them more challenging. There are also some new exercises for which you're definitely going to need your improved flexibility and your newly developed muscles.

Remember to read through all the instructions first before trying out a new exercise. Try one repetition and if it feels too tough, immediately look for a suitable modified version. Once you've mastered the simpler, modified version, then you're ready to move on to the unmodified one.

If any of the Level 3 exercises feel too difficult, if you feel any kind of ache or strain in your body, or have any injury or medical condition that prevents you from doing a certain exercise, just skip that one for now and return to it later when you are stronger and more flexible. Otherwise, keep to the order given as the program has been specifically chosen to give you a balanced workout.

remember the pilates principles

As you advance your practice, try to incorporate the six fundamental **Pilates principles** (see page 12) into your work. Each time you practice, pick one of them to focus on:

Breathing
Concentration
Control
Centering
Precision
Flow

As you get really comfortable and practiced at the exercises, you may want to pick up the pace a bit. Remember, Pilates is always about quality of movement. So never go so fast that you sacrifice the quality of the exercise, but if you're able to perform the movement well at a faster pace, then go on, challenge yourself a bit more.

Remember to use the transitions so that the exercises flow gracefully into one another so that the whole routine becomes one long, seamless movement.

Practice Pilates approximately thirty times and you'll feel you've got a whole new body—in fact, you will know you've got a whole new you.

level 3: exercise sequence char

This exercise sequence chart contains most of the exercises you learned in Levels 1

and 2, but some of them have been modified to make them a little more challenging.

There are also some brand-new exercises that will really change your body. As you

progress, remember to look back at the exercise instructions from time to time to make

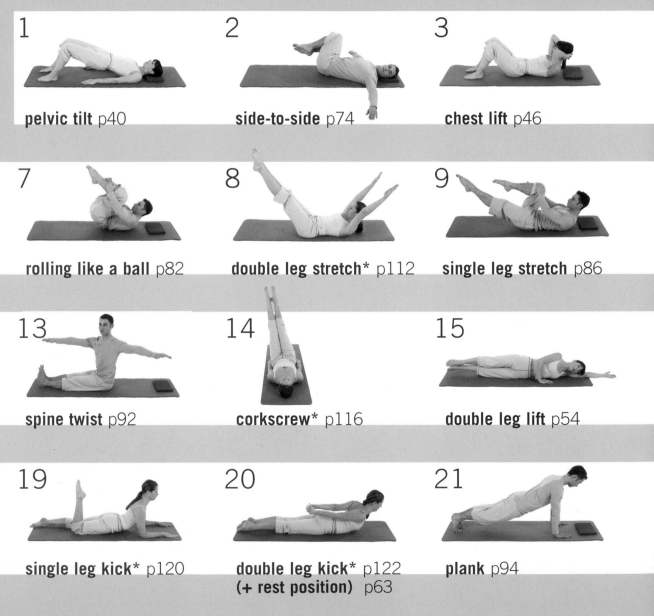

1
pelvic tilt p40

2
side-to-side p74

3
chest lift p46

7
rolling like a ball p82

8
double leg stretch* p112

9
single leg stretch p86

13
spine twist p92

14
corkscrew* p116

15
double leg lift p54

19
single leg kick* p120

20
double leg kick* p122
(+ rest position) p63

21
plank p94

* new exercises

sure you are still taking all the Precision Points on board, and also to see if you now

need to graduate to a more challenging modified version.

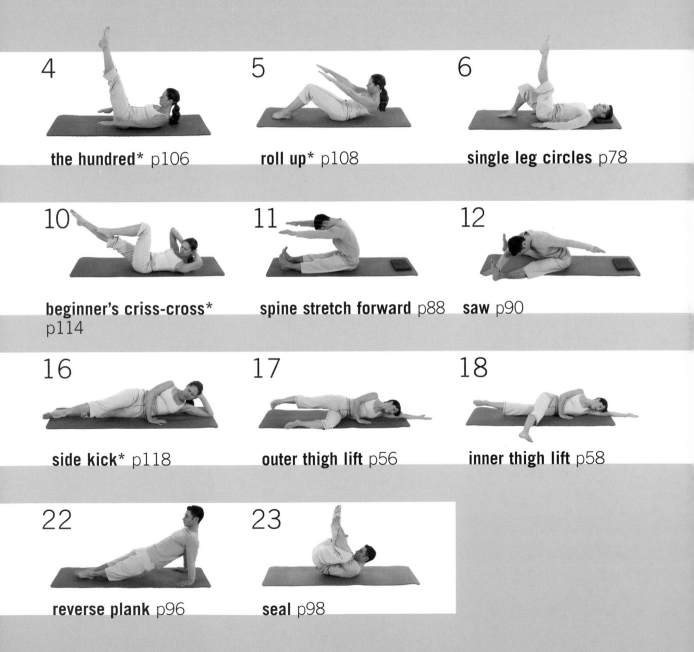

4 the hundred* p106

5 roll up* p108

6 single leg circles p78

10 beginner's criss-cross* p114

11 spine stretch forward p88

12 saw p90

16 side kick* p118

17 outer thigh lift p56

18 inner thigh lift p58

22 reverse plank p96

23 seal p98

the hundred

body benefits

- the ultimate abdominal strengthener

- strengthens upper back and chest muscles

- stimulates circulation

- builds stamina

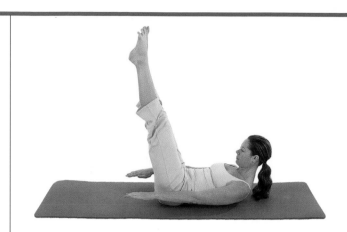

3 **Exhale**, drawing in the abdominals a little deeper, and stretch your legs up toward the ceiling. Keep the inner thighs glued together. *Imagine a heavy weight bearing down on your stomach as it sinks down toward the floor.* Look toward your navel.

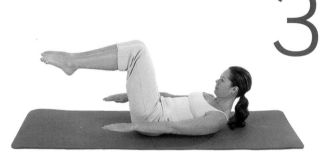

2 **Inhale**, keeping the abdominals engaged and initiating from them to roll your head and shoulders off the mat, hinging forward from the sternum. Stretch your arms away from you past your hips, keeping your shoulder blades down and your neck relaxed.

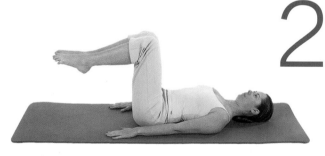

1 Lie on your back with your knees bent and your arms by your sides, palms down. Bend your knees in toward your chest. Lengthen the back of your neck and slide your shoulder blades down into your back. **Inhale**, then **exhale**, drawing in the abdominals.

precision points

✗

✗ **Don't lift your back too high off the mat.**

✗ **Don't allow your shoulders to lift up toward your ears.**

① ② **3**

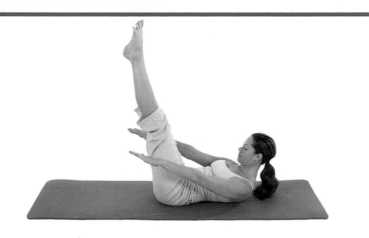

caution

● This is a tough exercise. If you feel any pain in your lower back, omit this exercise. If you feel tension in the lower back even when trying the modified version, omit this exercise until you can perform the exercise without arching your back or popping out your abdominal muscles.

4 Begin pumping your arms briskly up and down initiating from underneath the shoulder blades.

Inhale for 5 pumps and **exhale** for 5 pumps. Pump 100 times (i.e., 10 full breath cycles).

Transition: Draw your knees in toward your chest, rolling your head and shoulders down to prepare for the Roll Up (see page 108).

modifications

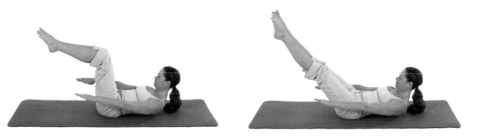

You may not be able to complete 100 pumps to start with. Begin with 50 and gradually increase the number of pumps each time you do the exercise.

If your back is arching or if there is any

tension in your lower back, bend your knees while you pump. Start to lengthen your legs to a 90-degree angle when you are stronger.

When you can comfortably perform the exercise with

straight legs, lower your legs to increase the level of difficulty. Gradually advance to a 45-degree angle.

If you feel any tension in your neck, just lower your head down and rest for a

while before trying again. If you still feel tension, take your hands behind your head and support the weight of your head in your hands while you stay in your position for the 10 breath cycles.

✓**Keep your back flat on the mat and your shoulder blades down throughout.**

✓**Ensure there is no tension in your neck. Think of hinging your body forward from your sternum, using your abdominals, not by pulling your neck forward.**

✓**Keep the pumps small and brisk, no higher than mid-thigh level. Keep your arms close to your body.**

✓**Breathe gently in through your nose and out through your mouth.**

roll up

body benefits

- strengthens the abdominal muscles

- stretches the back to improve flexibility

- encourages good spinal articulation

- lengthens the muscles in the back of the thighs

repetitions: 3–5

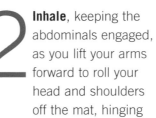

2 **Inhale**, keeping the abdominals engaged, as you lift your arms forward to roll your head and shoulders off the mat, hinging forward from the sternum. Make sure your shoulder blades are down and the base of your shoulder blades is still touching the mat.

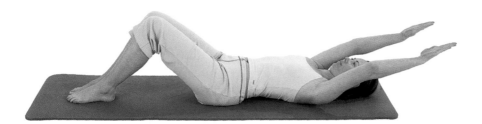

1 Lie on your back with your knees bent, feet and knees together. Reach your arms overhead, just above the level of your ears. Squeeze your inner thighs together. **Inhale**, then **exhale**, drawing in the abdominals.

caution

● Omit this exercise if you have any kind of back injury.

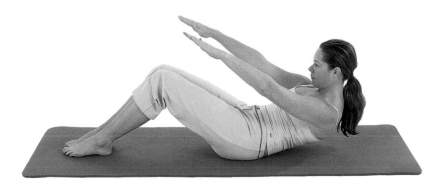

3 **Exhale**, drawing in the abdominals as you curl your body off the mat, peeling your spine off it one vertebra at a time. Try to create a letter C-shaped curve with your spine as you come up, pulling in your abdominals deeper and deeper the higher you come.

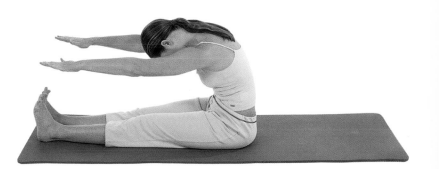

4 Keep rolling forward as you continue to **exhale**, rounding over with your arms parallel to the mat and your fingers in line with your ankles. Once your fingers reach past your knees straighten your legs with feet flexed as you continue to come forward. *Imagine you are rolling up and over a beach ball placed on your thighs.* Your will probably feel the stretch in the back of your thighs.

roll up cont.

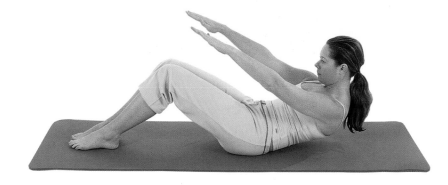

6 **Exhale**, drawing in the abdominals, and continue this flowing movement to roll your spine back down to the mat one vertebra at a time. Keep the C-shaped curve of your back throughout. You will feel your pelvis sliding underneath you as you roll back, and your shoulder blades stay down into your back. You are in Step 3 position again.

5 Reverse the movement. **Inhale** as you start to roll back until your shoulders are level with your hips. Slowly rebend your knees.

precision points

✗ Don't flatten your back; it should be in a C-shaped curve.

✗ Don't let your abdominal muscles pop out as you roll up.

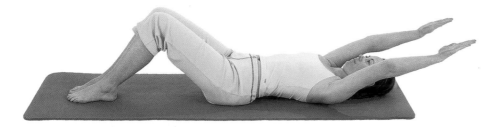

7 Once your shoulders reach the mat, continue to **exhale** and return your arms overhead, placing your head back down to return to Step 1 position. Repeat Steps 2–7 for repetitions.

Transition: Lower your arms to your sides to prepare for the Single Leg Circles (see page 78).

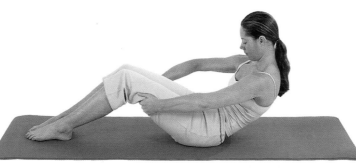

modifications

If you feel any tension in your back, or if you can see your abdominal muscles straining and popping out as you come up, crawl your hands up alongside your thighs to help you up.

If this still feels too difficult, do the Roll Down (see page 76) until you grow stronger and more flexible.

If you feel you are performing the Roll Up with ease, challenge yourself a little further by stretching both legs out in front of you for the whole exercise. Keep squeezing your inner thighs together throughout.

✓ **During Step 1, stay in neutral position. Be careful not to let your back arch or your ribs stick forward as you reach overhead.**

✓ **Keep your chin toward your chest and your shoulder blades down throughout. Don't use your shoulders to come up.**

✓ **As you stretch forward, keep the space between your hips and ribcage, so you are curved but not flopped.**

double leg stretch

body benefits

- strengthens the abominal muscles for a flatter, more toned stomach

- stretches the limbs for a more streamlined shape

- helps to improve circulation, reduce toxins in the body, and promote relaxation

repetitions: 5–10

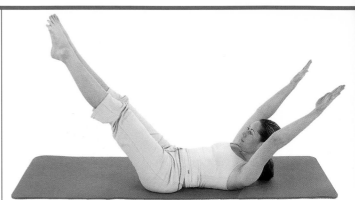

3 **Inhale**, keeping your abdominals engaged to support your spine, and stretch your body in opposite directions. Your legs extend to a 45-degree angle, while your arms lift straight behind you until they are in line with your ears. *Imagine your torso is glued to the mat as your limbs stretch away.*

2 **Exhale**, drawing in your abdominals, and roll your head and shoulders off the mat, sliding your shoulder blades down your back, your chin toward your chest. Feel your lower back lengthening along the mat.

1 Lie on your back and bend your knees in toward your chest. Your hands rest on your shins, elbows wide. **Inhale**.

precision points

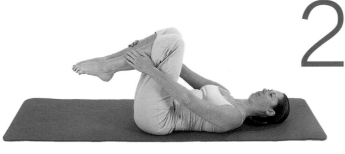

✗ **Don't lower your head and shoulders as you reach the arms back. Keep your chin toward your chest.**

✗ **Don't arch your back.**

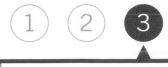

caution

● Proceed with caution if you have any back or disc injuries.

● Reduce the size of the arm circles if you have a delicate shoulder.

● If you feel tension in your neck, rest your head on your head rest for a few moments, or rest your head on a couple of pillows and perform the exercise in this position until you grow stronger.

4 **Exhale**, drawing in your abdominals again as you circle your arms out to the sides, then continue the circle to bring your hands back to your shins.

5 The legs bend back in at the same time so that you return to the starting position with your head and shoulders lifted and your hands resting on your shins (Step 2). Repeat steps 3–5 for required repetitions.

Transition: Lower your head and shoulders and bend your legs so that your shins are parallel to the mat to prepare for the Single Leg Stretch (see page 86).

modifications

If you find you are arching your back, or if you feel you are working into your lower back, lift your straight legs to a 90-degree angle so your toes point toward the ceiling to begin with. Gradually advance to a 45-degree angle as you get stronger.

✓ **Hold your straight legs strongly together by squeezing your inner thighs.**

✓ **Make sure your lower back remains on the mat throughout by using your abdominal muscles.**

✓ **Remain still in your torso. Only your arms and legs move.**

beginner's criss-cross

body benefits

- works the abdominal muscles

- trims the waist

- stretches the legs

repetitions: 5–10, alternating sides

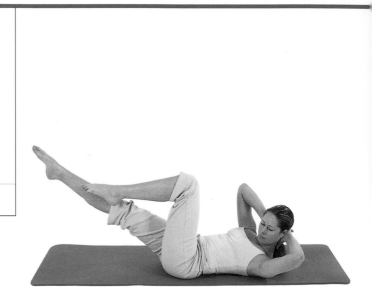

2 **Exhale**, drawing in the abdominals as you twist from your lower ribcage to bring one elbow over to the opposite knee. As you do so, straighten your other leg out to an angle of 45 degrees.

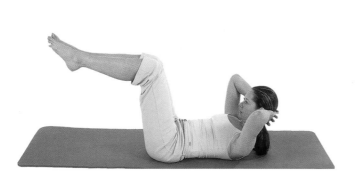

1 Lie on your back and bend both knees in so that your thighs are at a 90-degree angle to the mat and your shins are parallel to the mat. Interlace your fingers and place your hands behind your head.

Inhale, then **exhale**, drawing in the abdominals, to roll your head and shoulders off the mat, sliding the shoulder blades down the back. **Inhale**, keeping the abdominals engaged.

precision points

✗ Don't twist from your shoulders but focus on twisting from your lower ribcage.

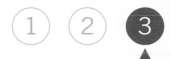

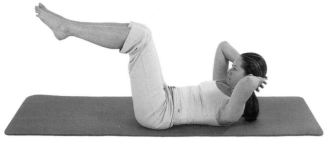

3 **Inhale**, keeping the abdominals engaged, as you twist from the lower ribcage to bring your torso back to center, bending your straight leg in again. Make sure your elbows stay wide throughout.

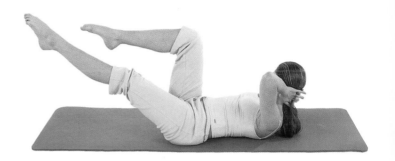

4 **Exhale** as you repeat but this time twist your torso to the opposite side, straightening the other leg. *Each time imagine your torso is staked to the ground so you don't rock from hip to hip.*

Transition: Bend both knees in toward your chest and lower your head and shoulders. Lower your feet to the mat with your knees bent at a 90-degree angle. Take your arms overhead and perform a Roll Up (see page 108) to bring yourself up to sitting in preparation for the Spine Stretch Forward (see page 88).

modifications

If this exercise feels difficult, lower your head back to the mat on each inhalation (Step 3) until your oblique muscles grow stronger.

✓**Keep your straight leg at 45 degrees. Don't let it sink toward the floor.**

✓**Keep your elbows wide so that they don't fold inward or touch the mat throughout.**

✓**Control the movement slowly and smoothly, don't just fling your upper body from side to side.**

corkscrew

body benefits

- strengthens the abdominals

- firms the inner thighs

- strengthens outer thighs and buttocks

- stretches the back

- improves balance

repetitions: 5 circles each side, alternating direction

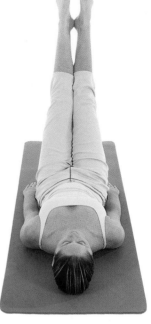

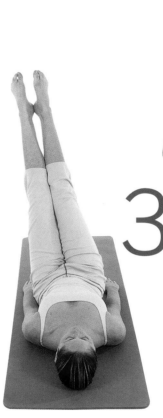

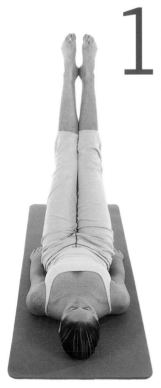

1 Lie on your back with your arms by your sides. Press your palms into the mat for extra stability. Lift and straighten your legs up to the ceiling at a 90-degree angle to the mat. Turn your legs out (see page 27), engaging your lower buttock muscles throughout. Your inner thighs will also engage.

3 **Exhale**, drawing in the abdominals, as you circle your legs down through the center line of your body.

2 **Inhale** and take your legs over to one side without allowing your body to lift. *Imagine your torso is rooted to the ground.*

precision points

✗

✗ Don't lift your hips and keep your lower back down on the mat throughout.

✗ Don't lift your shoulders or chin.

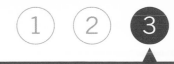
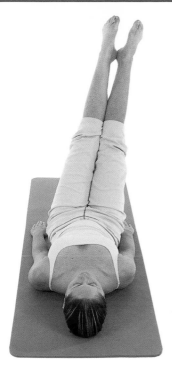

5 **Continue exhaling** as you circle the knees back up and in to the center. This movement is dynamic with the emphasis on the exhalation.

6 To reverse the movement: **Inhale** and take your legs over to the other side. **Exhale**, drawing in the abdominals, and circle your legs down, around, and back to the center.

Transition: Bend your legs in, then straighten them along the mat. Roll over to one side to prepare for the Double Leg Lift (see page 54).

4 **Continue exhaling** as you continue the circle over to the other side.

modifications

If your abdominal muscles pop out, or your back arches as you reach the low point of the circle, take your legs higher, until you are able to maintain your core stability.

As your technique improves, you can challenge yourself a little more by increasing the size of the circle without sacrificing stability.

✓Relax your neck and slide your shoulder blades down into your back to keep you stable as you circle your legs.

✓Think of reaching your legs up to the ceiling as you circle.

✓Circle your legs dynamically, with the focus on the upswing of the circle.

✓As you reach the lowest point in the circle, make sure your abdominals don't pop out, and your back doesn't arch.

side kick

body benefits

- tones the buttocks

- strengthens the hips

- trims the thighs

- streamlines your legs

repetitions: 10 each side

2 **Inhale** as you kick your top leg forward as far as you can without shifting your torso position. In this forward position, give a little extra beat at the top of the movement.

1 Lie on your side with one hip carefully stacked on top of the other. Your ear, the middle of your shoulder, and your hip and ankle should all be in a straight line. Your feet are pointing down. Now take your legs very slightly forward. Prop your head up on your hand making sure your elbow is in line with the rest of your body. Bend your upper arm and place your hand directly in front of you on the mat to help you balance. Make sure your shoulders are down and your neck is relaxed. Turn your legs out (see page 27) without moving your hips, engaging your lower buttock muscles. Lift your top leg a little so it is in line with your top hip.

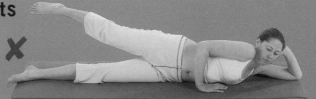

precision points

✗ **Don't allow your hips and shoulders to collapse forward.**

✗ **Don't allow your leg to lift above hipbone height.**

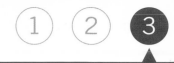

caution

● Proceed only under supervision if you have a neck or back injury.

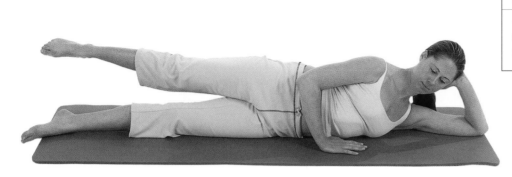

3 **Exhale**, drawing in the abdominals, keeping your legs turned out as you swing your top leg behind you, stretching the front of the hip. *Imagine your leg swinging like a pendulum.* Make sure you don't lean forward as you swing, and that your leg stays in line with your hip. Just swing your leg back as far as you can without compromising your torso position.

Transition: Bend your lower leg forward for the Outer Thigh Lift (see page 56).

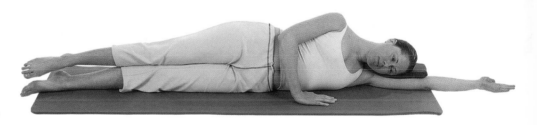

modifications

If you are rocking unsteadily so that you can't keep one shoulder on top of the other shoulder, and one hip on top of the other hip, reduce the size of the kick, until you become more stable.

If you feel any pain or tension in your neck or shoulders, or if you have delicate wrists or elbows, straighten your lower arm out along the mat and rest your head on top of it. You can even add a cushion between your head and upper arm for additional support.

✓ Keep the rest of your body completely still while you swing your leg back and forth, using your abdominals to keep your body stable.

✓ Be careful not to let your shoulders or hips move even a fraction forward or back.

✓ Keep your neck long and don't sink into your shoulders.

✓ Think of using your buttock muscles and the muscles in the back of your thigh to swing the leg back.

single leg kick

body benefits

- tones the back of the thighs

- stretches the often bulky front of thighs

- strengthens the back muscles

- stretches the front of the hips

- tones the arm and chest muscles

- increases spinal flexibility

repetitions: 6–10 each side, alternating sides

1 Lie on your front with your arms bent at right angles, palms flat on the mat. Your elbows should be positioned so that they lie under your shoulders, and your forearms should be parallel to each other and pressing into the mat. Lift your sternum and slide your shoulder blades down into your back. **Inhale**, then **exhale**, drawing in the abdominals, and keep your abdominals lifted throughout to protect your lower back. Squeeze your inner thighs together. **Inhale**.

precision points

✗ **Don't collapse your upper torso but keep your abdominals engaged throughout.**

✗ **Don't lift your shoulders.**

1 2 **3**

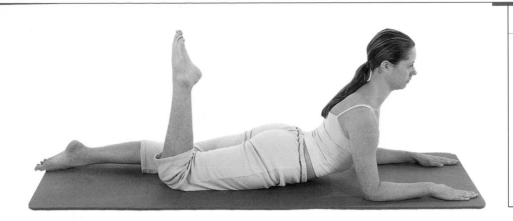

2 **Exhale**, drawing in the abdominals, and kick one leg toward your bottom, giving the leg a small extra beat at the top of the movement (near the buttocks). *Imagine you are trying to kick your buttock with your heel.*

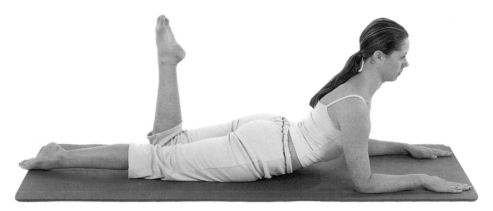

modifications

If the kicking motion brings on cramps in your hamstrings, reduce the range of movement and move more slowly.

3 Switch and kick the other leg toward your bottom, **exhaling** at the same time. Straighten the opposite leg when it is not kicking. The inhalation between the kicks is very small, almost a sniff.

Transition: Lower your head and shoulders. Turn your head to one side and take your arms behind your back to prepare for the Double Leg Kick (see page 122).

✓ Pressing your forearms into the mat and sliding your shoulder blades down your back will help keep you lifted.

✓ The exercise is most beneficial at a dynamic pace. To intensify, try not to place your leg down on the mat as your leg straightens; allow it to just hover above the mat.

✓ Feel your hamstrings working and your quadriceps stretching as you bend your leg, keeping your inner thighs and knees close together throughout.

✓ Lengthen through the back of your neck and focus your eyes straight ahead.

double leg kick

body benefits

- strengthens the back

- opens the chest

- increases spinal flexibility

- strengthens the back of the thighs and the buttocks

- stretches the often bulky front of thighs

repetitions: 5 each side, alternating sides

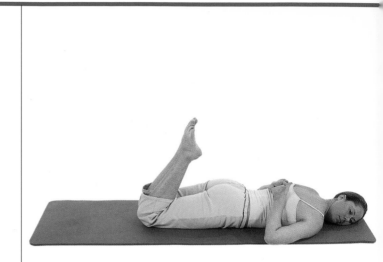

2 **Exhale**, drawing the abdominals in more deeply, as you squeeze your buttocks and inner thighs together. Kick your heels toward your buttocks three times. *Imagine you are a dolphin flicking your tail to swim.*

1 Lie on your front in a straight line, resting one cheek against the mat. Interlace your fingers and clasp them behind your back, taking them as close to your shoulder blades as is comfortable while still keeping your elbows and the fronts of your shoulders down on the mat. The palms face up to the ceiling.

Inhale, then **exhale**, drawing in the abdominals and then keep them lifted throughout the exercise. **Inhale**.

precision points

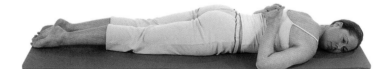

✗ **Don't lift your elbows and hips off the mat.**

✓ **Remember not to release your abominals when your lift your upper body, so that your spine is protected. You should not feel any tension in the lower back.**

① ② **3**

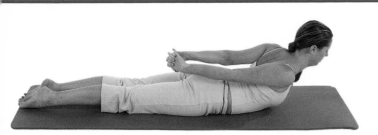

caution

● Omit this exercise if you have any kind of back injury or condition such as spondylolisthesis.

● Omit this exercise if you have problem shoulders or collarbones.

● Proceed with caution if you have delicate wrists, elbows, or knees.

● Stop if you feel any pain or tension in the lower back.

3 **Inhale**, keeping the abdominals engaged, and lift your upper body off the mat, and then straighten your arms and legs.

Focus your gaze straight ahead. Your hands reach away from you so that you can feel a stretch in your pectorals.

4 **Exhale** as you lower your body, bending your arms in again and turning your cheek. **Keep exhaling** as you bring your knees up again for the three little kicks. Repeat Steps 3–4 for required repetitions.

Transition: Roll up to a kneeling position, then sit at the front of your mat for the Seal (see page 98).

modifications

If you are unable to keep your elbows and shoulders touching the mat when lying flat, lower your clasped hands to the small of your back.

5 Sit back on your heels in the Rest Position for 30 seconds (see page 63) to give your lower back a gentle stretch.

✓Think more of smoothly lengthening your upper body away from your hips as you lift, rather than arching your back.

✓Keep the back of your neck lengthened as much as possible so that you don't crunch the back of your neck.

✓Focus on using the back of your thighs and your buttock muscles to make the three little kicks.

✓Make sure your legs and feet stay touching the mat while you are stretching your hands away from you past your buttocks.

continuing the journey

You made it. You've just experienced your first thirty Pilates sessions and are now fully aware of the power of this exercise method. You look better, you feel better, and you're undoubtedly hooked. Where do you go now to take it to the next level?

First of all, keep using this book. Keep practicing until you can perform all the exercises fluidly. Continue to focus on the six principles and on improving your technique. By the time you've mastered the exercises in this book, you are well into Intermediate Level.

finding an instructor

If you haven't already done so, it's a good idea to book a few private classes so that a qualified Pilates instructor can check on your technique and pinpoint any imbalances you may not yet be aware of, and give you guidance as to how to improve on these.

If you want your body to improve further, you'll then need to move on to the rest of Joseph Pilates' Intermediate Level mat exercises and then on to the Advanced Level mat exercises. It would be great to enroll in a Pilates mat-class and get some supervised instruction from a qualified instructor. Mat-classes are widely available. Before you select a mat-class, you need to check out a few things first. Find out how long your instructor trained for. Most good mat-training courses take about a year. Don't train with anyone who did a short course over a couple of weekends. Also, check out the size of the class. You really want a class of no more than twelve students. If the classes are too big, you won't get the supervision you are paying for.

the Pilates studio

You may also want to try taking classes at a Pilates Equipment Studio. Don't panic when you first enter one. Yes, it may look as though you've walked into a medieval torture chamber but rest assured that nothing painful goes on in there. In fact, it's hugely enjoyable and deeply relaxing.

In a Pilates Studio, the Pilates mat exercises are adapted so that they can also be performed on special machines that challenge your body to a different level. These pieces of equipment were originally designed by Joseph Pilates himself and possess intriguing names like "The Cadillac," "The Reformer," and "The Wunda Chair."

When you do your routine at home on the mat, you are using gravity and your own body to provide resistance. The Pilates equipment has ropes and pulleys and springs to provide even greater resistance, allowing your body to work harder, while improving alignment. Studio classes can be taken privately or semi-privately. Semi-private classes involve taking classes in small groups in which the instructor supervises each client while the client performs his or her own personalized routine.

Far more important than the various pieces of equipment in a Pilates studio, are the instructors themselves. Under the watchful eye of a good instructor, you will be guided through a program individually tailored to suit your strengths and weaknesses. Choose your instructor with care. As well as ensuring that he or she is properly qualified, you want to choose someone with whom you feel comfortable and able to ask questions of. Pilates is pretty hands-on and you want to be in a studio with an instructor who makes you feel relaxed, while challenging you to fulfill your body's potential.

Pilates will provide you with a lifetime of new challenges. You'll get the best body you can, improve your health, reduce stress, and feel younger and happier. The best bit about it is you can keep doing Pilates for the rest of your days. Pilates is a personal journey. Make it yours for life!

glossary

alignment
The position of the body in which the joints of the body are in line and symmetrical.

core strength
See *core stability*.

core stability
Also referred to as girdle of strength, core strength, or powerhouse, this is the band of muscles encircling the torso and extending from the lower ribcage to the pelvic floor, which need to be strong to provide stability or support for the spine.

draw in the abdominals
The drawing in of the abdominal muscles, in particular the transversus abdominis, and including the pelvic floor, to effect a hollowing in the waistline.

dynamic
The movement of one part of the body as a result of the amount of energy with which you perform it.

girdle of strength
See *core stability*.

leg turn out
The engaging of the buttock muscles to effect the external rotating of the entire leg in the hip joint. If you do this correctly, the inner thigh muscles will also engage.

lengthening
A visualization to induce stretching or straightening of a muscle without tension or strain.

metabolism
The rate at which your body burns calories. Your body will burn calories even when you are not moving. You can alter your rate of metabolism by increasing your lean muscle mass and by reducing body fat.

momentum
The force with which you exert movement. Your body should not be thrown around but moved with control.

neutral spine
Position in which the natural curves of the spine are present, and in which the pubic bone and two most prominent bones at the front of the pelvis (anterior superior iliac spine) are all on one level.

opposition
The act of using a muscle or muscle group in an opposing way to another muscle or muscle group.

Pilates box
Area defined from shoulder to shoulder, shoulders to hips, and hip to hip, to act as a reference for good alignment.

powerhouse
See *core stability*.

range of motion
The scope of movement within which a muscle can be safely exercised.

scoliosis
A curvature of the spine with a lateral curve one way and a rotation the other.

shoulder stabilization
The act of sliding or gently pressing the shoulder blades down the back, away from the ears, in order to put them into the best position for good shoulder and arm movement.

spinal articulation
The movement of the spine so that each vertebra moves individually and sequentially as you move through the spinal column.

synovial fluid
The body's version of lubrication for your joints. When you move, you increase synovial fluid production in your spine, hips, shoulders, etc. to keep them flexible.

visualization
The act of holding an image in your mind to help you recruit the correct muscles for an exercise or to help you perform it more fluidly.

index

acknowledgments

The author would like to thank the following:

Alan Herdman, Rael Isacowitz, and Anne-Marie Zulkahari for my Pilates training.

Huge thanks to Anne-Marie for her ongoing support and for being a constant source of inspiration.

The models—Pilates instructors Natasha Culmsee, Idris Moudi, and Lesley Pickering—for all their arduous posing under the hot lights.

Photographer Peter Pugh-Cook for the book's superb photos.

The team at Hamlyn, particularly Rozelle Bentheim for her creative direction, Geoff Borin for his design, Rachel Lawrence for managing the project, and my editor, Jane McIntosh, who suggested the book in the first place.

Wendy Rimmington and Suzannah Olivier for their help and encouragement.

And, of course, my husband for providing endless cups of tea throughout the whole process.

Executive Editor Jane McIntosh
Editor Rachel Lawrence
Executive Art Editor Rozelle Bentheim
Designer Geoff Borin
Senior Production Controller Jo Sim
Index Indexing Specialists

Special Photography Peter Pugh-Cook
Illustrations Bounford.com